A Natural Approach

Infertility and Reproductive Disorders

Macrobiotic Health Education Series

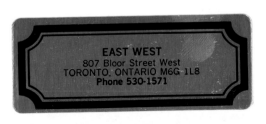

A Natural Approach

Infertility and Repro- ductive Disorders

by Michio Kushi

edited by Charles Millman and Phillip Jannetta

foreword by Christian Northrup, M.D.

Japan Publications, Inc.

Tokyo · New York

Note to the reader: Those with health problems are advised to seek the guidance of a qualified medical, or psychological professional in addition to that of a qualized macrobiotic counselor before implementing any of the dietary and other approaches presented in this book. It is essential that any reader who has any reason to suspect serious illness in themselves or their family members seek appropriate medical, nutritional, or psychological advice promptly. Neither this or any other health related book should be used as a substitute for qualified care or treatment.

Published by JAPAN PUBLICATIONS, INC., Tokyo & New York

Distributors:
UNITED STATES: *Kodansha International/USA, Ltd., through Harper & Row, Publishers, Inc., 10 East 53rd Street, New York, New York 10022.* SOUTH AMERICA: *Harper & Row, Publishers, Inc., International Department.* CANADA: *Fitzhenry & Whiteside Ltd., 195 Allstate Parkway, Markham, Ontario, L3R 4T8.* MEXICO AND CENTRAL AMERICA: *HARLA S. A. de C. V., Apartado 30– 546, Mexico 4, D. F.* BRITISH ISLES: *International Book Distributors Ltd., 66 Wood Lane End, Hemel Hempstead, Herts HP2 4RG.* EUROPEAN CONTINENET (except Germany): *PBD Proost & Brandt Distribution bv, Strijkviertel 63, 3454 PK de Meern, The Netherlands.* GERMANY: *PBV Proost & Brandt Verlagsauslieferung, Herzstrasse 1, 5000 Köln, Germany.* AUSTRALIA AND NEW ZEALAND: *Bookwise International, 1 Jeanes Street, Beverley, South Australia 5007.* THE FAR EAST AND JAPAN: *Japan Publications Trading Co., Ltd., 1–2–1, Sarugaku-cho, Chiyoda-ku, Tokyo 101.*

First edition: February 1988

LCCC No. 85–080533
ISBN 0–87040–638–8

Printed in U.S.A.

Foreword ━━━━━━━━━━━━━━━━━━━━━━━

The ability to conceive and bear children is a natural function that is often taken for granted. And the desire to "participate" in future generations by producing offspring is as ancient and instinctive as the human race itself. Yet, the number of couples facing infertility is increasing each year.

The anguish associated with this problem is tremendous. It is not at all unusual for one or both members of the couple to feel guilty, often resulting in marital discord. As the couple's stress levels increase, chances for conception can be further decreased.

For many, intervention, in the form of a support network, is extremely important, so that the individuals no longer feel so ostracized, isolated, and different from others. Networks, such as "Resolve," exist nationwide, lending support to individuals and couples.

Infertility is often complex, involving not only each member of the couple but their combined interaction as well. Modern medicine tends to focus on the physical body when making a diagnosis. But the emotional and spiritual aspects of the individual and couple are equally important. The relatively new field of *psychoneuroimmunology* lends tremendous support to the ancient concept of emotions and thoughts creating either health or disease.

The holistic approach to health-care encourages people to take responsibility for their dis-ease or health. In treating infertility, it is important that each individual or couple follow a course of action that feels appropriate for their stage of development. Very seldom is infertility a clear-cut problem requiring simple correction. Most often, changes are needed on several different levels. Clearly, improving nutritional status cannot be over emphasized. A diet high in complex carbohydrates, rich in trace minerals, and low in fat, can go a long way toward normalizing hormonal and physical functioning.

In addition to a healthful diet, it is important that individuals become mindful of their bodies through regular exercise or movement. Our society is so fast-paced that most people must consciously and intentionally learn to "tune-in" to how their bodies are feeling. It is astounding how many people have no idea what a relaxed body feels like. Chronic misuse of, and lack of attention to, our body's wisdom can result in subtle hormonal dysfunction as well as other illnesses.

The work of Thomas Verney, M.D., David Cheek, M.D., and

others documents the role of emotional blocks in infertility. Sometimes, for example, deep-seated subconscious trauma from one's own birth or childhood will predispose to infertility. It is important that infertile couples take steps to dissolve these blocks. For many, the use of acupuncture, Feldenkrais, music or art therapy, or a number of other body-centered modalities can be extremely helpful. Remember that 20 percent of all infertile couples have what is known as "medically unexplained" infertility. And many formerly "infertile" individuals, with medically documented causes for their problem, have gone on to conceive with different partners or when other circumstances in their lives have changed. Given this, we encourage couples to seek not only competent medical care but also to look beyond the "medical model" in their journey through this distressing time.

Finally, the experience of physical infertility affects how fertile one feels in the world. The importance of this cannot be over-emphasized. Whether or not a child is eventually born, the experience of being or having been infertile can have lasting impact on one's life. Optimal "recovery" from infertility in the broadest sense means feeling fertile and creative on all levels of life, including career and relationships.

May this book be a signpost along the way to helping you reclaim your birthright of optimal health of body, mind, and spirit.

Christiane Northrup, M.D., FACOG
Marcelle Pick, R.N.C., M.S.N.

Introduction ▬▬▬▬▬▬▬▬▬▬▬▬▬▬

Humanity's primary orientation, like that of all biological life, is the survival and development of the species. However, in modern times, we are trying to accomplish this strictly through material gain and material power extending far beyond what is necessary. In other words, men are using their traditional role as provider and protector for excessive mastery over nature, and to build a societal structure that greatly exceeds natural needs. With this orientation, men have created the class systems, educational systems, legal systems, and engineering and technological systems. And, men have followed this path to instigate history's wars as well.

Until the beginning of the Industrial Revolution, women generally were not as involved in building these institutions. Since that time, however, women have begun to compete with men for position and power. As a consequence, the central biological position of women as nourisher and keeper of the species has begun to collapse.

These two trends have resulted in a growing frustration of both sexes. Thus, it has become necessary to explain the nature of men, and the nature of women, and the dynamics of their relationship, from the wide perspective of the macrobiotic principles.

Modern science and medicine, with their increasing dependence on high technology, are bringing about the emergence of an artificial species. Through the disappearance of natural human qualities and functions, comes a distortion of the species—even though we maintain our human form, we are becoming non-human. This new, weakened species, will collapse before the middle of the next century, even if we do not have World War III. Indeed, this impending collapse is the most pressing problem humanity now faces.

A sign of this degeneration and degradation is the extent to which men and women are losing their unique qualities. Impotence and infertility occur much more frequently today than even thirty years ago. A host of male disorders, including prostate problems, weak or no sperm, and high blood pressure, combined with the epidemic of women's reproductive problems (hysterectomies, ovarian cysts, chaotic menstruation), reflect the diminishing of the natural human being.

Most of this degeneration can be blamed on the interrelated factors of poor eating habits and imbalanced psychological conditions. Our modern way of life, including diet, disrupts the vitality of the male and the female reproductive systems. The resulting lack of physical strength, energy, immune ability, and basic fertility, can be expressed as a loss of the power of species survival; a loss of the sustaining power of the human spirit.

The challenge we now face is twofold: 1) How to recover natural fertility and natural survival ability, and 2) How to reverse the degeneration of humanity in modern society. Modern science and medicine are not the answer. Collectively, their approach is characterized by artificiality, thus advancing our unnatural status.

We must, then, use natural ways to recover and strengthen our original biological strength. This means that we adopt a balanced diet and lifestyle, as outlined in this book.

In addition, men must become physically active. We should discipline ourselves to exercise regularly, so that natural energy can flow freely and smoothly. And, we must learn to use our bodies more in daily life, instead of depending on mechanical devices.

Women, too, should make every effort to improve their health, especially their reproductive functions, which are central for the creation of new life. The unique ability of women to give birth and nourish their children is, in reality, the determining factor in our planet's future. From this perspective, the greatest gift a mother can give her children is health, because health allows her offspring to develop infinitely in whatever direction they choose.

Gradually, as lifestyle and diet change, natural human reproductive power will return. This is the only way the human species can secure its basic human spirit.

I hope that is book, along with its companion volume in the *Macrobiotic Food and Cooking Series*, will contribute to the reversal of the modern trend toward reproductive decline, and the re-establishment of natural human fertility.

I would like to thank all of the people who contributed to the publication of this book, including our associates Charles Millman and Phillip Jannetta, for compiling and editing the material for this work. I thank our friends and associates at Japan Publications, Inc., Mr. Iwao Yoshizaki and Mr. Yoshiro Fujiwara, respectively president and New York representative, for their guidance and advice. I thank Edward Esko for his assistance and dedication. I also thank Jay Kelly for contributing the artwork and illustrations, and Judy Pingryn, of Becket, Massachusetts, for her work in typing the text. I also thank Helaine Honig for her efforts in compiling Avelin Kushi's companion volume, *Cooking for Infertility and Reproductive Disorders*.

Contents

1. Infertility: A Macrobiotic View ▬▬▬

> Not having a baby is torture. The worst God-awful punishment
> that I could imagine. Everytime I go to the store or drive down
> the street and see a woman pushing a baby carriage, I feel like
> I'm nothing, just worthless. It is especially bad when I meet
> someone I know with a child. I think, why can't that baby be
> mine? What did I do?
>
> My husband doesn't want to go out. We just stay at home
> night after night. I know no one would say anything, at least
> not intentionally, but I can see that look in their eyes, almost hear
> that unasked question. I used to cry all the time, but now I guess
> I know. We will keep trying. Maybe a miracle can happen. I just
> wish I knew why. I would almost have anything else than this.
> Really. I know it sounds strange, but I would if I could just have
> a baby.

This woman's anguished words help personalize the terrible impact
infertility and reproductive disorders inflict on both men and women.
One of humanity's basic biological functions, procreation, is only
a dream for her and her husband. And, as more and more people are
learning, reproductive disorders are far from rare. The number of reported cases is increasing dramatically, although until recently, the
problem has been cloaked in an almost embarrassed silence.

If there is one thing each of us takes for granted, it is our own
reproductive ability. Having children is looked upon as an inherent,
God-given right. Sadly, this is not the case for one out of every five
couples in the United States today. Thus the explosion of information
on infertility and reproductive disorders in recent years.

Reproductive disorders have become one of the hottest topics of the
1980s. The media—national and local—have helped bring this issue
to public attention. Newspaper and magazine articles and features,
radio and television talk shows, documentaries, and news specials
are driving home both the extent and the impact of the problem.

The following quotations will help put perspective on the situation:

New Conceptions by Lori B. Andrews, F. D.
William Mosher of the National Center for Health Statistics
recently compared two surveys—one taken in 1965, the other in
1976—that are the most recent attempts to assess infertility on a
national level. He found an 83 percent increase in infertility among

married couples in which the wife was between 20 and 25 years of age, traditionally a most fertile group. The 1976 survey found that about 10 percent of all married couples were infertile. Now the figure is estimated to be about 15 percent.

The actual figures for infertility are much higher than that, claims Martine O'Connel, chief of the Fertility Statistics Bureau of the Census Bureau. "These surveys label infertile a married woman who has tried to have a child in the past year and failed. But there are many women who are infertile and just don't realize it yet because they haven't tried to have a child."

Diet and Disease by Cheraskin, Ringsdorf and Clark

The exact incidence of involuntary sterility is difficult to determine. Vital statistics provide a record of births in relation to marriages and to population, but do not distinguish the failure to conceive from the accidents of early pregnancy, and take no account of the use of contraception. A conservative analysis of the best available data indicates that somewhat more than 12 percent of modern marriages are barren. There are, in the United States today, nearly 3,000,000 childless couples who are still at the age of potential reproduction.

Time

Infertility, which now affects one in six couples, is on the rise. According to a study by the National Center for Health Statistics, the incidence of in fertility among married women between the ages 24 to 29, normally the most fertile age group, jumped 177 percent between 1965 and 1982.

Cosmopolitan

Like the growth in primary infertility, there has been an increase in the number of couples with secondary infertility. These people come from all races, all religions, and all economic backgrounds.

MS

Medical experts estimate that more than ten million people, one out of every five couples in this country, have some kind of infertility problem, and the numbers are growing.

Newsweek

At least 10 million American men, one out of every eight, are afflicted with the agony, frustration, humiliation of impotence.

"Be fruitful and multiply" was one of the first commandments God gave to mankind. The continuation of the human species has been assured because we have been able to do just that. This fertility is a reflection of humanity's overall health and vitality, and specifically, of the health and vitality of our reproductive system. By any standard, however, out general health in modern society is declining, and this trend is reflected in the weakening of our reproductive functions.

Limiting our focus to infertility and reproductive disorders alone fails to convey the scope of our overall decline. Reproductive disorders are part of a pattern, a much larger pattern, unfolding in this country and in many other industrialized nations. A look at a brief health profile of the United States will give us an idea of how healthy we are as individuals and as a nation.

Currently, the major diseases that afflict us, and our leading causes of death, are of the degenerative nature. By definition, degeneration means: "A lowering of effective power, vitality, or essential quality to an enfeebled and worsened state." It is worth noting that this definition can apply equally to degeneration of the physical, emotional, intellectual, and spiritual realms. And this is exactly what the leaders of our major social institutions—education, religion, economics, and the judicial system—are warning us about.

A more specific definition of degeneration is: "Deterioration of a tissue or an organ to the point where its function is diminished or its structure impaired." Thus, in degenerative disease, the very structure and functions of our body's systems, organs, and cells are eroding. This is a frightening thought, and yet there is scarcely a family that has not been touched with some form of degenerative disease, as the following statistics reveal:

Cancer: According to the latest studies, one out of every three babies born in 1985 will have cancer in his or her lifetime. This compares with one out of fifteen in 1950. In 1985 alone, an estimated 910,000 people were diagnosed as having cancer.

Arthritis: Currently 50 million Americans—every fourth person— have some form of arthritis. This includes more than 7 million crippling cases. *Osteoarthritis*, or degenerative joint disease, affects 97 percent of all people over 60.

Diabetes: Diabetes currently ranks as the seventh leading cause of death in the United States. It claims over 340,000 lives each year, and over twice that many new cases are reported annually. One out of every four American babies born in 1984 is expected to develop diabetes in his or her lifetime.

Cardiovascular disease: Cardiovascular disease is the number one cause of death in the United States (and in most industrialized countries). It affects an estimated 40 percent of the U.S. population. According to the American Heart Association, medical expenses and lost productivity due to heart disease cost the nation an estimated $64.4 billion in 1984.

As most of us are probably aware, the rate of incidence of each of these degenerative diseases continues to climb. What we may not realize is that these disorders are not confined to the elderly. The fact is that increasing numbers of middle-age and young adults suffer from degenerative disorders. And worse, there is a long list of other illnesses that testify to the declining quality of our health: Epilepsy, 2.1 million cases, or 1 in every 100 people; Allergies, 39 million cases, or 1 out of every 6 people; Alcoholism, an estimated 14 million cases, or 1 out of every 10 adults; Mental illness, at any given time, 29 million Americans, almost 1 out every 5 adults, suffer from psychiatric disorders ranging from mildly disabling anxiety to severe schizophrenia.

The impact of these and other health problems on the economic and social viability of the United States is massive. And in each case, the pattern is the same—there is a large-scale incidence that continues to climb.

The second category in our health profile deals with hospitalizations. This is determined by recording the total number of hospital discharges, and the average length of stay of patients from short-stay institutions.

Discharges from non-Federal short-stay hospitals:

Patients under age sixty-five:	
All discharges:	27,898,000
Average length of stay:	5.9 days
Patients over age sixty-five:	
All discharges:	10,697,000
Average length of stay:	10.1 days
Total number of discharges:	38,593,000

The fact is, we in this country are requiring more frequent visits to the hospital, and longer stays, than ever before.

The last factor we will consider in this health profile of the United States is the cost of health care. (Figure 1)

Fig. 1   Health Care Costs in the United States

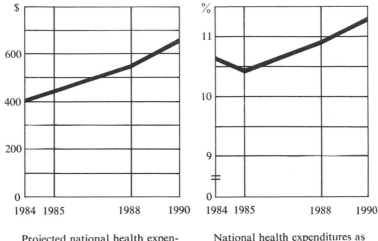

Projected national health expenditures in billions of dollars

National health expenditures as
a percentage of GNP

National health expenditures for 1985 are projected to be over
$400 billion. This figure will have consumed more than 10 percent of
our Gross National Product (GNP)—the total value of all goods and
services produced in a year. Figure 1 vividly illustrates the continu-
ing climb in our medical bills if the present trend of sickness is not
altered. By 1990, that is, in just three years, our health expenditures
will be over $600 billion, a figure representing more than 11 percent
of the GNP.

As increasing numbers of medical procedures based on high technology come into routine use, the cost of both testing and treatment
will rise sharply. Because we are sick more often, because we are more
likely to suffer from degenerative disease requiring extensive treatment
and more frequent hospitalization, and because our on-the-job productivity is being negatively affected, our nation's total fiscal resources are being squandered. Several obvious conclusions can be
drawn from this brief health review.

1.   The overall health of this country is declining at an alarming rate.
The strength and vitality of our biological bodies, and thus our
ability to function normally, is eroding. During our lifetime, the
chances are that most of us will suffer from at least one major degenerative disease.

2.   The financial burden of this problem is saping our economic

resources as increasing amounts of our money must be diverted from other, more productive areas, to pay our health-care costs. Being sick is expensive. And the financial strain it puts on those who are healthy, and whose taxes pay a large portion of these health costs, is growing.

If this decline in public health continues, the economic integrity of the nation must also decline. Or, put another way, the continued existence of the United States (and other modern countries) as a vital national entity, is in jeopardy. Consider what will happen over the next decade as productivity continues to decline because of workers' poor physical and/or mental health; as the amount of work days missed due to illness continues to increase; and as the number of disabled workers temporarily or permanently removed from the work force climbs. What is at stake, in reality, is the continuation of society as we know it.

As the above trends continue to grow, there will necessarily be sharp changes in the way our country functions, and in the way we as individuals and families live. No society can withstand the steady erosion of its wealth, vitality, and productivity. Thus, three major developments seem to be emerging to counteract these trends.

1. *The mechanization of the work force.* This process is already well under way, and refers to the use of machines, and more recently robots and computers, to replace humans in the workplace. Initially, the rationale for this transition was to relieve humans of monotonous or dangerous work. Now we hear about the dependability and efficiency of the machines, and of more leisure time for workers.

One of the basic principles of macrobiotics is that every front (obvious or positive side) has a back (hidden or negative side). In the recent bestseller, *The Reckoning*, author David Halberstam discusses the impact that the automated assembly line had on the automobile industry and the general public. Mass production reduced costs and greatly increased output. Company profits soared even as prices dropped, making it possible for the average American to purchase a car.

In the next section, Halberstam tells us how the assembly line changed the workplace. "These new jobs demanded much less skill and offered much less satisfaction. Men who had prided themselves on their skills and had loved working with machines found themselves slaves to those machines, their skills unsummoned. The machines, they discovered to their rage, were more important than they were."

As machines become increasingly sophisticated, humans will be relegated to tasks requiring little if any skill or physical effort. Pride of work, creativity, and sense of job fulfillment will vanish. In addition, special hospital-like environments will be needed to bring the increasing numbers of disabled individuals back into the work force.

2. *The mechanization of human beings.* This development involves the introduction of mechanical and manmade parts into the human body. Examples include artifical blood, skin, organs—hearts, kidneys, livers, lungs—inner ears, limbs, and joints. As daily news reports attest, this alternative is well under way, and with full government support, is rapidly progressing.

3. *The creation of replacement organs through high technology and genetic engineering.* Although not yet practical, researchers the world over are racing to develop marketable devices. Included in this category is the creation of artificial life, that is, life created in a laboratory. The technological tools to accomplish this seem to be available. Already, for instance, genetically engineered bacteria have been developed and, supported by a court order, have been tested in the open air. Experiments with higher forms of life continue.

Certainly, most people would choose normal, natural health to any of the three alternatives above. And it is a choice we are all being given. We can accept responsibility for our personal well-being or we can put ourselves into the hands of the health-care industry. Our increasing rate of serious disease, coupled with the rapidly developing bio- and medical technologies, are creating fundamental issues of human health and morality to be decided by each one of us.

Infertility and Reproductive Disorders ——————

As we have shown, infertility and reproductive disorders cannot be separated from the overall trend toward biological degeneration; as one declines, so must the other. One major fertility clinic in Britain, for instance, discovered that 30 out of 100 men (their wives were being treated at the clinic) suffered from previously undetected health problems ranging from high blood pressure and diabetes, to chest tumors and skin disease. The same clinic found that nearly all its female infertility patients who required surgery for blocked tubes or other pelvic adhesions also had a heart murmur, or *mitral valve click*. In one study, they found that 100 out of 125 women who had some form of pelvic adhesions also had a heart murmur.

Current statistics on infertility are grim. According to a 1982 study published by the National Center for Health Statistics, during the period from 1965 to 1976, there was a 65 percent increase in infertility among couples where the wife was between the ages of 15 and 28. These are the prime child-bearing years for women.

The study also reported that as of 1976, there were 4.3 million married couples, or 1 out of 6, with infertility problems. However, the study did not include single or divorced persons, and did not count as infertile any of the estimated 19 percent of the couples who were using some form of contraception. A certain portion of these people can be expected to be infertile.

Some experts now estimate that as many as 8 million couples in the United States are infertile. Of course, this figure does not consider the numerous men and women who have put off marriage in order to pursue careers. A certain percentage of these individuals may also be infertile.

These findings, and others like them, make it clear that infertility, and reproductive disorders that can lead to infertility, fit into the trend of declining health established earlier in our health profile.

Current Approaches

A couple consulting a physician on the suspicion that one or both partners might have a fertility problem will undergo a series of tests as the first step in their treatment. Because tests to determine infertility in women are complex and expensive, a man will usually be examined first.

The list of possible tests for men, after a complete medical history and a thorough physical, can include analysis of the semen and sperm —their quantity, shape, and motility—a *vasogram* X-ray, biopsy of the testes, urine and blood tests, hormone-level check, and sperm antibody test.

For women, after the medical history and physical, tests can include basal body-temperature charting, pelvic examination, analysis of cervical mucus, endometrial biopsy, urine and blood tests, post-coital test, *hysterosalpingography* (an X-ray study in which radio-active dye is injected into the uterus to show the outline of the uterus and the degree of openness of the Fallopian tubes), and *laparoscopy* (direct examination of the ovaries, Fallopian tubes, and uterus with an instrument inserted through a small incision in the abdomen). The extent of these tests can depend on the judgment of the physician and the patient's condition.

Individually, or as a group, these tests can be painful, expensive, and time-consuming. They invade into the intimate lives of the individual or couple, and are often seen as humiliating. In addition, test results often do not yield the concrete answers the couple seek. But, as one man asked, "What are my alternatives?"

After the test results are in, various drugs could be prescribed. In an attempt to elevate male sperm counts, for example, *clomiphene citrate, human menopausal gonadotrophin*, or *human chorionic gonadotrophin* may be recommended.

For women, clomiphene citrate is used to stimulate the release of the hormones *follicle stimulating hormone* (FHS) and *luteinizing hormone* (LH). *Pergonal* is used to stimulate the ovaries so that a follicle grows to maturity. Human chorionic gonadotrophin (HCG) is used to bring about ovulation. (Both pergonal and HCG are derived from female urine.) Other drugs may include *gonadotrophin release hormone*, which stimulates the pituitary gland; *bromocriptine*, which reduces elevated prolactin levels; and *danazol*, to treat endometriosis.

These are not the only medications used. A complete list is beyond the scope of this book. However, it must be pointed out that the drugs listed above, like all drugs, have side effects that must be carefully monitored.

If drug therapy is not called for, or if it fails to help, surgery may be the next available step. Depending upon the problem, any of a variety of surgical procedures could be performed on either the man or the woman. Examples include removal of blockages, scar tissues, adhesions, and tumors. Laser surgery and microsurgery have made the outlook for such treatments brighter. But if the surgical alternative is not called for, or if it proves unsuccessful, the couple might consider—as more and more couples are—one of the new technologies to achieve a pregnancy.

Technologically Assisted Conception

Call them what you will—a miracle of science or a perversion of nature—the age of technologically assisted methods of conception is upon us. And despite the fact that they are provoking a storm of controversy—religious, moral, and legal—research and implementation are going on around the world.

Artificial insemination (AI) is the oldest of an expanding inventory of treatments using high technology to overcome infertility. This procedure involves the introduction of sperm into a woman's uterus or vagina by mechanical or instrumental means to increase the likelihood of conception. If the husband's sperm is inadequate, a third party or *donor sperm* could be used. If the wife is incapable of carrying a baby, the husband's sperm could be introduced, in ways mentioned above, into another woman, who would carry the baby for the couple. This arrangement is called *surrogate mothering.*

In-vitro (test tube) *fertilization* (IVF), is another of the new fertility techniques. The first so-called test-tube baby was born in 1978, and hundreds have since followed. *In vitro* refers to a biological reaction occurring in a laboratory apparatus. In this process, fertilization takes place in a laboratory dish instead of a woman's womb. After conception, the fertilized egg is implanted in a woman's body. Depending on the cause of the problem, the following possibilities exist for In-vitro fertilization: wife's egg or donor's egg; husband's sperm or donor's sperm; wife or a substitute mother carries the baby. Also participating are the doctors, nurses, and lab technicians. Sexual intercourse, the most private and personal of acts between two people, has become in effect, a group effort, and a state-of-the-art medical procedure.

We must remember, however, that procreation assisted by high technology did not come about by chance. A problem existed, namely infertility, and researchers worked to alleviate it. In other words, we as individuals have allowed our condition to deteriorate to the point that science and technology were asked to come to the aid of one of our basic human functions. In the years to come, we can expect the necessity for such treatments to rise, and the complexity of the technology used to become increasingly elaborate.

The problem of infertility itself, our increasing dependence on the products and procedures of biotechnology, and the startling capabilities that are emerging in this field, present grave implications both for individuals and for society.

Social Implications

"Are we going to set up a market, if we go the frozen embryo route?" asks a professor of health at Boston University. "Should that become the norm? Should embryos be merchandised like Cabbage Patch dolls? What will that mean in relationships between mother and child? What are the implications for the family structure?"

The basic unit of society is the family. It is humanity's oldest and most durable institution. The family, quite simply, is the foundation upon which civilization is built. One primary function of the family is to create healthy children, and to give those children a sound physical, mental, and spiritual orientation so that they will become self-sufficient members of society. The ability to accomplish this is based on a common biological link and the shared experiences of its individual members. Today, with the use of fertility technologies, the family's common biological link is being severed.

It is within the family unit that the basic teachings of human values and behavior takes place. Infertility threatens the continuation of the family and its role as the primary institution in human society. What is unfolding, in effect, is the erosion of civilization itself.

In this century the family has already undergone drastic changes. Until relatively recently, the primary family structure was the *extended family*. By definition, extended families consist of several generations living in the same household. Most often this includes grandparents, parents, and children, and perhaps grandchildren, cousins, aunts, and uncles. In industrialized societies the extended family has been replaced by the *nuclear family*, made up of parents and children.

Currently, the nuclear family is losing primacy as increasing numbers of couples—for various reasons—do not have children, and as more and more *single-parent families* appear. The causes for the later phenomenon are varied, and include divorce, premature death of a spouse, and single parenthood. Both trends, however, are symptoms of broader social, economic, and biological influences which will be touched on later.

Now, with the increasing rate of infertility, family life seems to be undergoing a new mutation: the specter of the *artificial family* looms on the horizon. It is here that the common and unifying biological inheritance, passed from generation to generation, is being broken. We face the stark and very real possibility that the biological family, as a group united by common blood and genes, will lose its dominance.

Ethical Implications———————————————————

As we have seen, fertility disorders are forcing increasing numbers of couples to choose the alternatives offered by modern science and high technology to realize their dream of having children. This can produce a moral dilemma, because many religions do not approve of such techniques.

The Roman Catholic Church, for instance, strongly opposes artificial insemination by anyone other than the husband. This stance was first articulated in 1949 when Pope Pious XII decreed: "Artificial insemination in marriage, but produced by the active element of a third person is . . . immoral and, as such, to be condemned." The Lutheran Church, most Anglican Churches, and Orthodox Jews also oppose artificial insemination by a donor. Protestant and Reformed Jewish groups generally approve, although there are dissenters.

Aside from religious conviction, scientific methods of conception raise basic ethical questions for individuals and society as a whole. What is the proper role of science in creating human life? Where are the boundaries beyond which technology should not step? Or, indeed, should restrictions be applied to an area of research and application that promises to relieve a variety of health concerns?

When the basic impulse to have a child is denied through natural methods, a couple can face agonizing decisions. Should they remain childless, or should they try to adopt a child—a difficult, expensive, and time-consuming process. Or, in spite of any religious or ethical misgivings, should they attempt to achieve a pregnancy through technological assistance. These and other moral issues will confront a growing number of couples in the years ahead.

Legal Implications

What happens when a surrogate mother decides to keep the child she has contracted to carry for another couple? This was a matter of judicial speculation, until just such a case reached the courts recently causing a storm of accusations and controversy. Law makers and judicial experts agree that our legal system is not prepared to deal with this and other new realities created by the emerging application of science to the creation and manipulation of human (and also plant and animal) life.

What happens, for instance, when an anonymous sperm or egg donor wants to contact his or her offspring? Or when an artificially conceived child asks to meet his or her biological father or mother. Increasingly, our overburdened courts will be forced to deal with these and related issues. Experts foresee an entire new field of law emerging, and the passage of extensive and complicated legislation. We can also expect a heated debate as governmental agencies are forced into a role unimagined just one or two generations ago.

Health Implications

Humanity has taken a step into the darkness with the advent of artificial methods of fertilization. We have no way of knowing what the long-term effects of these new technologies may be. Equally disturbing is the fact that technicians, in the absence of guiding principles beyond the concept that if a thing is possible it should be done, seem to be making basic decisions concerning crucial human issues. By default, they are preempting the role of religion, philosophy, and government. History and experience point out the dangers of such an approach. When a group with specialized interests—whatever their intentions—are free to make decisions affecting broader social issues, tragedy is in the offing.

There is another, obvious danger as well. "Look before you leap" is a bit of folk wisdom that can be applied to every area of human affairs. Increasingly in the twentieth century this bit of common sense has been disregarded, resulting in unparalleled misfortune for modern society. But nowhere is this lesson being violated with more impunity than in the treatment of infertility.

Too often, so-called miraculous medical, scientific, and technological innovations have been prematurely made available to the general public. Then, as the full implications of these innovations have emerged, they have been withdrawn or outlawed. Just one example is the drug *thalidomide* which in the 1950s was prescribed for pregnant woman suffering from morning sickness. Too late, it was discovered that the medication created devastating birth defects in the children of the women who used it.

Who takes responsiblity in such cases. Who can compensate a child born without legs or arms. Who can comfort the parents of such children. In this instance, the drug was withdrawn and, despite public outcry, the issue was allowed to fade without broad public, scientific, ethical, and legal debate of the tragedy's larger implications. If we do not learn from our mistakes, we will certainly be forced to repeat them.

What qualities are lost, diminished, or added, when sperm and eggs are removed and then reintroduced into the human body. What are the effects when they are frozen in liquid nitrogen at minus 196°C., and stored for future implantation. What happens when conception takes place in a laboratory dish and the fertilized egg then implanted, sometimes after being stored for weeks, months, or longer. Do we have the answers to these questions. Is anyone even asking. And, finally, where is the broad perspective that can consider the myriad of implications involved—moral and ethical, biological and legal.

In our desperation to prevent or resolve basic biological degeneration, have countless couples become willing partners in the gravest experiments in humanity's history. Have the offspring of such couples become unconsenting subjects, being forced to pay the price of their parents inability to maintain health, and science's eagerness to extend its mastery over natural processes. In chapter 2 we will look at the process of conception and of sexual intercourse from a broader perspective.

Personal Implications ─────────────────────

Perhaps no affliction causes more distress than infertility. Despite ever-changing social values, the impulse to create children and a family remains deep and strong. Yet, as we have seen, millions of men and women are unable to do so. The number of infertile couples is large and increasing rapidly. Cases of infertility have doubled in just the last ten years. "Infertility has reached epidemic proportions," admitted one researcher.

The inability to have a child places tremendous emotional and mental pressure on a man and/or a woman. It can lead to the questioning of one's personal worth as a human being. Individuals may begin to wonder, "What is wrong with me? What did I do wrong? What is my value?" Thoughts of worthlessness, guilt, and failure are common.

The damage to an individual's self-image can lead to strong, even violent emotional reactions. These tensions can easily destroy a relationship and spill over into all areas of an individual's life. An individual may even decide that life is no longer worth living.

The Cause of Infertility ─────────────────

Both infertility, and reproductive disorders that can lead to infertility, are essentially physical health problems. The implication is that humanity's deep-seated biological integrity is eroding. Because of this overall degeneration, it would be a mistake to narrowly focus attention in our search for solutions.

The symptomatic approach to health problems, or to any concern, can be misleading, frustrating, and even dangerous. Trying to understand body parts and functions apart from their relationship to the whole, and isolated attempts to correct problems that affect them, is impossible. Admittedly, short-term, symptomatic relief may be found, but this is achieved at the cost of long-term well-being. Simultaneously, such an approach implies the abandonment of the search for practical methods of prevention. What happens in this case is that we end up treating the results or effects of a problem, while allowing the underlying cause to go unchecked. And because the cause goes untreated, new and more serious symptoms usually emerge.

This approach is something like turning off a ringing fire alarm in the middle of the night and going back to bed. The disturbing symptom, the noisy alarm, has been relieved, while the cause, the fire, is permitted to continue its damaging and life-threatening course. Obviously, no one would do this. And yet, in a very real sense, this is precisely the course we are pursuing in our approach to physical health.

Common sense tells us that there are specific reasons for any changes in the body's functions and structure. Our inability to discover these reasons is more a commentary on the effectiveness of our approach than on the absence of understandable causes. A basic premise of science, one that seems forgotten by many scientists, is that there is a cause for whatever happens, and that a cause will in turn produce effects. We may not understand the reasons, but we sense they are there to find. The implication is clear: for permanent relief of undesirable effects, the cause must be discovered and eliminated.

Despite what we may have been taught, our bodies are not self-contained entities, existing independently from our physical and social environment. We are in constant interchange with our environment, near and far. Cold and heat, light and dark, sound and sensation, the lunar cycles, the rhythm of the seasons, even magnetic storms on the far-off sun are examples of the multiple external factors that create internal bodily responses. There is a ceaseless interchange going on between our internal and external environments. Our *physiology* is a complex set of checks and balances that maintains equalibrium between the two.

Of all the processes by which we internalize and adjust environmental factors, eating is by far the one we have the most control over. In modern society the word diet has taken on narrow and negative associations. It calls to mind images of deprivation, will power, and unreasonable sacrifice. The macrobiotic definition is much different.

We start by realizing that food refers to anything that we take in. This of course includes the solids and liquids that we consume at mealtimes. It also embraces the air we inhale, the sensory stimulation we absorb through our nervous system in the form of touch, smell, taste, hearing, and sight. Food further includes the enormous range of vibrations that we constantly receive from our immediate environment and from the far reaches of the universe.

In the largest sense, our diet includes all of these, and dietary practice can be seen as the attempt to create harmony within and between each category. An additional aspect to the meaning of dietary practice is the conscious attempt to adjust our food to create the type of physical, mental, and spiritual qualities we desire.

Clearly, our level of control over food, in its largest sense, varies widely. By the wise choice of our daily food and drink, however, we influence all aspects of our life. For instance, respiration and heart beat vary in response to the quality and quantity of what we consume. Hormone levels and blood-sugar levels, nerve impulses and reaction times, perspiration and urination levels all vary in response to what we are eating. Emotional and mental states, as basic parts of our self, are also directly affected by daily diet.

The link between diet and physical health has been established. There are too many studies, from too many reputable sources, for this fact to be denied. A look at current recommendations of various health-related associations, including the American Heart Association, the American Diabetes Association, and the American Cancer Association, confirms this. In addition, reports issued by governmental agencies—*Dietary Goals for the United States*, issued by the U.S. Senate Committee on Nutrition and Human Needs; *Healthy People: The Surgeon General's Report on Health Promotion and Disease Prevention;* the National Academy of Sciences' report, *Diet, Nutrition and Cancer;* and the Canadian and British dietary guidelines —move this fact beyond the realm of debate. It only remains for governmental and professional policy, and awareness among the general public, to come to terms with the implications. The next major area of investigation, which is now actively going on, is the link between emotions, behavior, and food.

Few of us appreciate the crucial role food plays in our lives. And yet the fact is confirmed from whatever view we approach it—biochemical, physiological, economical, or simply from the perspective of common sense. Our body, including the nervous system and brain, is originally created directly by the foods our mother eats during pregnancy. (Even more basic, the quality of our parent's reproductive cells, before conception, was influenced by the nourishment they consumed.) This process continues after birth with food providing the materials for an infant's rapidly growing body. Following physical maturation, the body constantly renews and repairs itself, again from daily food and drink.

Cultures around the world and throughout history have recognized this essential function of daily food. In fact, many have deified their primary food. Regional cuisines have developed in response to local environmental conditions. That is to say, a sophisticated body of knowledge of local foods, their uses and effects, was developed and passed from one generation to the next. Each cuisine has a well-developed understanding of medicinal foods, specific recommendations for pregnant women, growing children, and the aged.

Traditional religions, almost without exception, have taught dietary recommendations to the general public. They have offered special practices for days of celebration and for days of ceremony. For individuals seeking spiritual development, specific dietary suggestions were given.

It should be now clear that the starting point in the investigation of any health problem should logically be the day-to-day diet of the individual concerned. Specifically, infertility and reproductive disorders are primarily the result of the kinds and amounts of food an individual has been eating, and the effects of these foods on his or her body and mind.

Illness of any sort represents the body's natural adjustment to an improper or inbalanced diet and lifestyle. The key to reversing an illness is to make order in these areas. Lifestyle is a factor too often overlooked in the healing arts. Our daily activities can either aggravate a condition, or if properly used, be a powerful tool in maintaining or recovering health and vitality.

Within the category of diet, two possible sources of trouble exist. The first is the eating of improper foods, that is, foods which do not contribute to health and which may detract from it. The second is eating in excess, even good-quality foods. In combination, these factors can be deadly. Our bodies cannot efficiently digest, assimilate, or metabolize foods in the improper category. Nor can the body eliminate such items through normal channels of discharge—urination, exhalation, perspiration, bowel movement, and so on.

As a result, residue, in a form that is often toxic, begins to build. Initially, this happens in more peripheral areas as the body attempts to localize, neutralize, and discharge them. Over time, and with continual abuse, these processes are either overwhelmed or depleted, and excess begins to accumulate deeper within the body. This marks the beginning of various cysts, tumors, tissue build-up, chemical and hormonal changes, and organ degeneration that lead to, among other things, reproductive disorders.

Modern Diet

An obvious question needs to be answered at this point: What is it, exactly, in our dietary practice that we are doing wrong?

Macronutrients is the name given to the group of three nutrients humans need in the largest amounts. Taken in descending order of amount required, these include carbohydrates, protein, and fat. The average American diet is composed of approximately: 40 to 50 percent carbohydrate; 40 to 50 percent fats; and 10 to 15 percent protein. To fully appreciate the consequences of such an eating pattern, we must examine it both in terms of quality and of amount.

1. Carbohydrates are often referred to as sugars, and as carbohydrates come in a variety of forms, this can be a source of mis-

understanding. Simple sugars or *monosaccharides* and double sugars or *disaccharides* bypass the body's complex system of digestion and absorption. They move quickly into the bloodstream, giving one a burst of energy, causing an overacidic condition, and raising blood-sugar levels. To balance this condition, the pancreas secretes *insulin*, a hormone which brings high blood-sugar levels down by enabling excess sugar in the bloodstream to enter body cells.

For optimum health, the intake of simple and double sugars should be drastically reduced or completely avoided. Common forms include cane sugar (*sucrose*), milk sugar (*lactose*), fruits (*fructose*), honey, and maple syrup.

A third type of carbohydrate or sugar is complex sugar or *polysaccharides*. Complex sugars are digested gradually, and enter the bloodstream at a slow, steady rate. They provide a constant source of energy over a relatively long period of time. Equally important, complex carbohydrate foods—grains, beans, and vegetables—also contain a variety of other nutrients including oils, proteins, minerals, and vitamins which both help in the metabolism of complex carbohydrates and provide extra nutrition. (For a complete discussion of carbohydrate metabolism, please refer to our book, *Diabetes and Hypoglycemia* in the *Macrobiotic Health Education Series*.)

Since the primary function of carbohydrate is as an energy source, the quality of the carbohydrates we consume plays a vital role in our physical, mental, and emotional vitality. And by any measurement, we consume far too much simple sugar, if indeed there is any safe level.

2.   Protein is primarily used to build muscle and organ tissue, and to replace worn out tissues. The body also uses small amounts of protein to manufacture hormones and enzymes. There is some controversy over the amount of protein needed on a daily basis, although many experts agree that Americans consume excessive quantities. In addition, we tend to consume animal-quality protein, which is high in saturated fats, as well as in the growth hormones, antibiotics, and other medications that are fed to animals. All of these substances are passed on to those who subsequentally eat the animal products. In the words of one doctor:

> Animals ingest antibiotics, chemicals, and hormones. When we eat meat (or dairy food), we are nibbling on everything the animals eat. Short of becoming vegetarians, we cannot avoid eating a variety of compounds that are added to our meant. It is a troubling realization.

3.   Fat is used by the body basically to store reserves of energy. However, when fat is burned as energy, it produces toxic wastes that must be neutralized. This is one reason why there is general agreement that our diets contain far too much fat.

The fat we consume is usually of the saturated variety, derived from animal sources including beef, pork, poultry, eggs, and dairy foods. In nontechnical terms, saturated fats are more difficult for the body to break down and use. Instead of being properly metabolised, they are deposited throughout the body. Excess fat, especially saturated fat, is stored in and around the blood vessels and body organs, including the reproductive organs, and is the leading cause of infections, tumors, cysts, and cancer in these areas.

Excess or poor-quality fat has the additional effect of blocking absorption of digested foods by the intestinal villi, absorption of oxygen in the lungs, and the elimination of wastes by the kidneys. It also can block skin pores, thus interfering with the skin's respiratory and discharge functions, and with the circulation of environmental energy.

One final point is worth mentioning. If we experience an immediate reaction (within a few hours or perhaps the next day) from something we eat, say a headache or upset stomach, vomiting or diarrhea, we know the cause was what we ate, perhaps in combination with the amount consumed. The relationship is clear. To prevent similar problems in the future, we simply do not eat that particular food, combination of foods, or excessive amounts again.

Often however, our reaction to an unbalanced or poor-quality food is less pronounced, perhaps not even noticable beyond a certain lack of energy or a somewhat dulled thinking. Many people have abused themselves for so long, that their sensitivity and discharging systems no longer function properly. This is unfortunate, because these individuals miss the connection between what they are eating and the quality of their health, days, weeks, even years later. Then, when their sexual appetite diminishes, tumors form, tubes are blocked, or sperm count drops, they fail to recognize the actual cause of the problem, concentrating instead on symptoms.

There is a consciousness gap that must be bridged. The length of time it takes before problems make themselves known through strong symptoms can be quite long. However this does not alter the fact that such a condition has been developing for an extended period of time, perhaps many years, and that the cause lies in our daily lifestyle, particularly in our day-to-day diet.

Understanding Health ─────────────────────────────

Someone once remarked that frequent public discussion about a value or virtue is a sure sign that that particular quality is in short supply. In recent years there has been an explosion of discussion on the topic of health. As the quality of national health declines, increasing amounts of time is spent discussing it. But what does the concept really mean.

The dictionary defines health as: the condition of being sound in body, mind, or soul. The implication is that our physical body—cells, blood, organs, nerves, systems, and so on—is functioning properly, that is, without the need for artificial or extraordinary support. In addition, our emotions are stable, and our mentality clear. Interestingly, included in this definition is the soul, which can be expressed as the harmony of physical and mental functions working smoothly and efficiently.

Actually, this is a suprisingly broad definition, one each of us would do well to consider. It implies that health is a dynamic interaction of all aspects of our selves—physical, emotional, mental, and spiritual. By extension, it suggests that if there is a problem in one area, the whole will be affected. If a physical problem develops, for instance, there will be a corresponding emotional and mental reaction.

It is easy to overlook the holistic or ecological relationship of our existence. Too often we think of problems as separate concerns, having no connection to our physical body as a whole, or to the other aspects of our self. If a man is experiencing trouble with his sperm quality, for example, he and his physician are likely to concentrate on the specific factors that influence sperm production. It is likely that the man's overall physical condition, if it falls within certain parameters, will be ignored as a contributing factor. This approach does not represent a total health strategy, nor does it reflect a comprehensive understanding of health and sickness. The major defect in this piecemeal approach is that it fails to address the basic problem. Certainly symptoms may be relieved, but others will develop until the cause is eliminated.

The Emotional/Mental Connection ───────────────

When a physical complaint arises, we quickly become aware of our biological existence. Too often, however, we fail to recognize our associated mental and emotional imbalances. Perhaps we no longer worry about them, attempt to ignore them, or at best, view them as separate problems. But as we have seen, there is an emotional/mental side to any sickness. If we suffer from constipation, for instance, it is doubtful that we are happy-go-lucky. Clearly then, the mental and emotional aspects of infertility and reproductive disorders are as important as the physical ones.

Emotions and mentality fluctuate according to the state of our physical health, and in response to external or environmental circumstances. Where then does the basic source of these fluctuations lie? Every experience, whether perceived as positive or negative, elicits an emotional/mental response. The appropriateness of our response is our concern here. If, for example, someone criticizes our work, we react. Our response could be anger, resentment, self-pity, despair, and so on. Or, we could reflect on the comment to determine if it is valid. If so, we have gained an opportunity for self-improvement. If not, the individual has given us insight into his or her own character and state of health.

Some days it is easy to remain cheerful and optimistic. On others even the slightest thing may set us off. Do we ever stop to consider why. If so, we probably mumble something about being in a bad mood, needing a vacation, or something similar. The key to our emotional/mental response is the quality of our biological health. When it is sound, the functions and reactions of our total body are balanced.

The fact is, we are not brought up with the expectation that we can discover the cause of our mood swings, of our health problems, and of the direction that our life is taking. These things just happen, and if they become unbearable, we engage an expert to relieve the symptoms.

It is a terrible mistake to diminish the importance of working with the mind and the emotions when trying to change a physical problem. By using methods to enhance these aspects of ourselves, we can greatly increase our chances of recovery and accelerate the process. Such practices can also be used, like physical exercise, as a means to establish well-being and continual growth.

In our efforts to temporarily (symptomatically) cope with mental and emotional problems, we reach for tranquillizers, sedatives, antidepressants, and other drugs that alter our moods. But this is not the answer. These substances prevent real growth, eliminate symptoms while masking the cause, and often produce dangerous physical and emotional side effects. More natural, holistic alternatives include prayer, meditation, self-reflection, activities that encourage self-expression, visualization, breathing exercises, massage, physical activity, and increased contact with nature. Along with dietary change, these practices help us fashion a total program for health. We are using all aspects of our being.

Consciousness—the combination of our emotional, mental, and spiritual selves—is capable of bringing about fundamental changes in our body. In fact, this is happening all the time, for better or worse, sometimes slowly, in other cases very rapidly. Proper diet strengthens the biological source of these abilities.

Most of us have read or heard stories of almost miraculous recoveries brought about by the application of the powers of the mind. Actually, this is only the most dramatic part of the story. What is missing is the obvious but seldom made acknowledgment of the dynamic interaction of the whole body—physical, mental, and spiritual. These stories do, however, demonstrate the ability that is in each of us to help ourselves.

Macrobiotics: A Dietary Philosophy

Although macrobiotics is commonly thought of as a diet, it can more accurately be called a dietary philosophy. It is a comprehensive approach that, under different names, has enabled civilizations to flourish in their particular environment and historical period.

The basic premise of macrobiotics is that there is a universal order that governs all life and all phenomenon. This pattern is called the Order of the Universe and its principles are based on the observation that:

1. The universe and everything in it are in a continual state of change.
2. Human beings are not exempt from this pattern.
3. There is an understandable order to this change.
4. We have only to understand and live in harmony with this order to ensure the health and the full development of each aspect of our selves—physical, mental, and spiritual.
5. Traditional religions, moral and ethical teachings, customs, myths, arts, and so on, represent regional interpretations of this order.

The Unifying Principle is the name given to the forces that govern this pattern of change. It is based on the complementary and opposite nature of the universe. All phenomenon, from a preatomic particle to the motion and structure of distant galaxies, are governed by two opposite yet complementary tendencies. These tendencies are called *yin* and *yang* (traditional Oriental terms) in macrobiotic philosophy.

Yin refers to the centrifugal or expanding tendency, or movement away from the center. Yang refers to the centripetal or contracting tendency, or movement toward the center.

Applied to food, this concept implies that any particular food item has one of either two general effects on our body, mind, and spirit —either contraction or expansion. A partial listing of various complementary characteristics found in food is included below.

	Centrifugality—yin	Centripetality—yang
Size	Expanded (large)	Contracted (smaller)
Shape	Leafy	Root
Color	Purple, green	Brown, orange, red
Region of growth	Warmer	Cooler
Season of growth	Summer, spring	Fall, winter
Rate of growth	More rapid	Slower
Category	Fruit, vegetable	Bean, grain
Liquid content	More moist	Drier
Sodium content	Less	More
Taste	Pungent, sour, sweet	Salty, bitter
Cooking required	None, less	More

Using the Unifying Principle, we can devise a chart showing the yang or yin effects of various foods, and the relative strength of each. This is represented in Figure 2. The farther from the center we go in either direction, the stronger the yin or yang effect.

The application of this understanding is what is called the macrobiotic approach to diet. It is important to realize that rather than being a diet in the contemporary sense of the word, this is a way of living based on natural and universally applicable principles. Thus within broad general guidelines, an individual's way of eating will vary according to age, condition, occupation, locale, and future goals. It will vary from season to season, and to a lesser degree, from day to day.

The macrobiotic approach to diet, besides pointing out what foods should be consumed, and in what relative amounts, also stresses the importance of proper cooking, manner of eating, and the understanding of the energy our foods provide.

Because of the limitless scope of the Order of the Universe, the macrobiotic principles can be applied to any topic or question we wish to study. This provides a deeper insight into the basic nature of life.

Figure 2 helps convey the breadth of application of the Unifying Principles of change. Within each category, we could also create

Fig. 2   General Yin (▽) and Yang (△) Categorization of Food

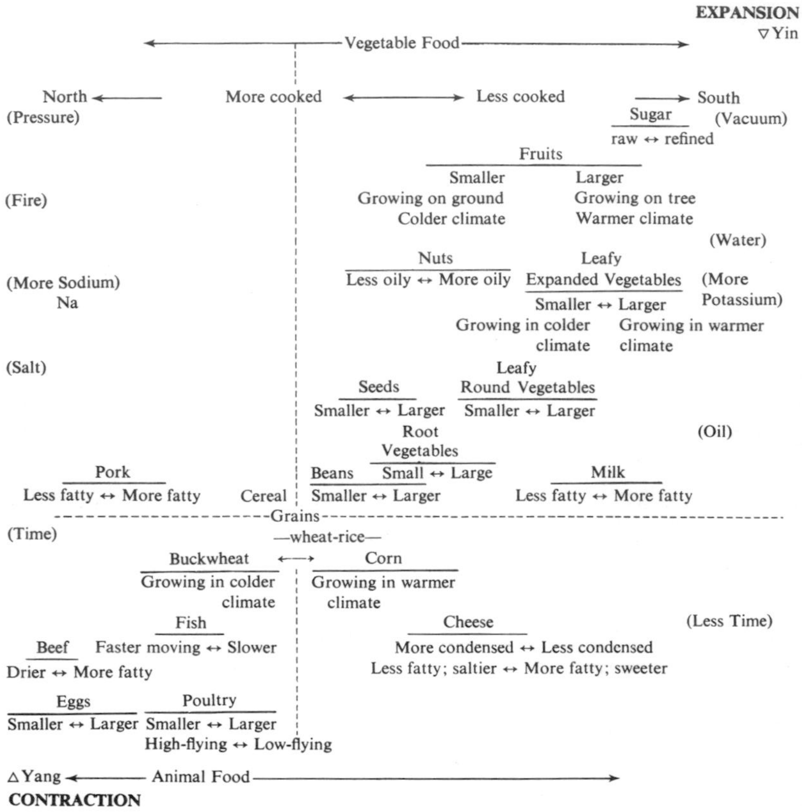

EXPANSION
▽Yin

◄————————— Vegetable Food ——————————►

North ◄——————   More cooked ◄————————► Less cooked   ——————► South
(Pressure)   Sugar   (Vacuum)
                                                                  raw ↔ refined

                                                          Fruits
                                              Smaller   Larger
(Fire)   Growing on ground   Growing on tree
                                      Colder climate   Warmer climate
                                                                          (Water)

                                        Nuts   Leafy
(More Sodium)   Less oily ↔ More oily   Expanded Vegetables   (More
  Na   Smaller ↔ Larger   Potassium)
                                                     Growing in colder   Growing in warmer
                                                          climate   climate

(Salt)   Leafy
                                         Seeds   Round Vegetables
                                    Smaller ↔ Larger   Smaller ↔ Larger
                                                         Root   (Oil)
                                                      Vegetables
            Pork   Beans   Small ↔ Large   Milk
  Less fatty ↔ More fatty   Cereal Smaller ↔ Larger   Less fatty ↔ More fatty
(Time)   ------------------Grains--------------------------------------
                                    —wheat-rice—
                Buckwheat ←——→   Corn
                Growing in colder Growing in warmer
                    climate   climate
                  Fish   Cheese   (Less Time)
    Beef   Faster moving ↔ Slower   More condensed ↔ Less condensed
  Drier ↔ More fatty   Less fatty; saltier ↔ More fatty; sweeter
    Eggs   Poultry
  Smaller ↔ Larger Smaller ↔ Larger
                    High-flying ↔ Low-flying

△Yang ◄————— Animal Food ————————————————————————►
CONTRACTION

The above chart gives the general classification of food groups from yang to yin. However, more precise classification should be made upon examination of environmental conditions, nature and structure, chemical compounds, and effect upon our physical and mental conditions. Also, cooking can greatly change food qualities from yin to yang and yang to yin.

more specific yin and yang tendencies. For a more detailed view of yin and yang tendencies, please refer to any of the variety of macrobiotic books explaining how the concept can be applied to individual topics.

Yin and Yang ———————————————————

As we have seen, the universe is governed by the ceaseless interplay of two fundamental tendencies—yin and yang. Examples include day and night; full moon and new moon; summer and winter; male and female; youth and old age. The list is endless, and the pattern is everywhere the same: yin or expansion changes into yang or contraction, and then, at its extreme point, reverses direction again.

Although this change is an inherent aspect of all phenomenon, the rate varies from thing to thing. In some instances it is incredibly fast—from our point of view—like the life span of certain insects. In others it is so unimaginably long that we may tend to think of it as eternal—the lifetime of a star is an example. Both examples, however, the insect and the star, have a beginning and an end, and move from one to the other through a recognizable pattern of development. Only their scale in time and space differs.

Nothing is exempt from the principle of change, nothing exists outside the realm of yin and yang. In the countless examples we encounter everyday, from our swings in mood and energy levels, to changing weather patterns, yin and yang reveal the basic principles of life.

The Spiral of Life

The universal order that is found on every level of existence is revealed in the multidimensional form of the logarithmic spiral. This form clearly conveys the basic truth of existence: On a fundamental and undeniable level, we are unitied with everyone and everything in the universe.

Most of us have seen photographs of spirally formed galaxies, and perhaps we have noticed some of the many spirals found in the human body—the hair spiral on the back of the head, or the spiral on our finger tips, for example. From the growth of plants, to the movement of ocean currents, the spiral is the basic pattern of life. It is the spatial representation of yin and yang in motion. Certain things may not constitute a complete and perfect spiral, but this is because they are either forming or disintegrating. If our view is wide enough, we will recognize the spirallic pattern and motion in all things, and in all dimensions of life.

Yin and yang, and the logarithmic spiral, are the basic tools of macrobiotics. They enable us to reconcile apparent contradictions, and solve all mysteries in life. Thus there is a macrobiotic approach to any field we care to deal with, including medicine, nutrition, spiritual studies, economics, the sciences, and so on.

The basic pattern of the universe has been recognized, articulated, and applied throughout human history. Its understanding is part of our heritage as human beings, and is actually nothing more than common sense.

As mentioned previously, civilizations have recorded this comprehension in various ways, including architectural structures, agricultural traditions, and ancient calenders. One the clearest examples of this traditional understanding comes to us in the form of humanity's timeless teachings. Although the method of expression varies to suit unique environmental and historical periods, the underlying concept is the same.

The Bible offers countless examples of the complementary/opposite nature of reality. In the *Book of Genesis*, creation is described in terms of darkness and light, heaven and earth, land and water, for example. In classical Indian literature of the *Vedanta*, in the mythology of American Indians, in ancient Egyptian, Roman, and Greek legends, in Buddhist and Taoist literature, the basic teaching is the same; life moves in alternating currents which are reflected in the lives of individuals and civilizations.

The Macrobiotic Way of Thinking —————————

How is it that in our modern world, with our wealth of scientific and technological breakthroughs, the concept of yin and yang is not to be found. The answer lies in our orientation to life. Since classical Grecian times we have increasingly tried to uncover nature's secrets by searching for the basic building blocks of life. Our approach has been to continually refine our techniques for analyzing and breaking down. As our tools have grown more sophisticated, our view has narrowed. Modern science and technology is now characterized by specialities and sub-specialities. We are attempting to understand the nature of reality by going ever inwards. Recently, however, modern physics, the mother of all our sciences, tells us that at the subatomic level, we have reached the limit of our narrow focus. From this point, existence expands into waves of energy.

As a result of our analytical approach, we view things as separate and isolated, and assume that we can deal with individual parts with no recognition of the relationship of the parts to the whole. To verify this view, an incredible number of divergent hypothesis have been put forth to explain various phenomenon.

A hypothesis is designed to explain a particular set of data. If a hypothesis is proved, it becomes a theory. Yet although theories determine our approach to various questions, no theory is ever absolutely and finally proved. Theories can exist for thousands of years, and then suddenly fall to new data and new hypotheses. The theory that the earth was the center of the universe was suddenly destroyed by Galileo. Today, countless assumptions that we take as certainties, are just as susceptible to sudden reversal.

Clearly, modern society lacks a unifying principle that will explain and harmonize life into a comprehensive ecology of existence. We are drowning in an excess of facts and details, or knowledge, and parched for an overall operating orientation, or wisdom.

Macrobiotics offers humanity the key to unraveling life's mysteries. It provides a comprehensive orientation that recognizes the interdependence of all life, and gives us an understanding of our origins and our destiny. Reproductive disorders take on a new meaning when studied with the Unifying Principle of yin and yang. Their causes and course of development become understandable, and natural methods for relief suggest themselves. Before looking specifically at such problems, however, we will take an overall look at the human body, and see how the reproductive system functions in harmony with the whole.

2. The Reproductive System———

From the macrobiotic perspective, any discussion of infertility and reproductive disorders (or any health problem) must begin with an understanding of the body as a whole. The insights this wider view provides can then be practically applied to the specific topic of the reproductive system. As mentioned earlier, the tools we use to gain this perspective are the Unifying Principles of yin and yang, and the logarithmic spiral.

The yang force, motion, or tendency originates in the farthest reaches of the universe, and spirals in toward the center of the earth. Its major entrance points are the north and south magnetic poles. The effect of this motion is contraction, fusion, and solidification. In more poetic terms, yang motion is called Heaven's force, that is, the force or energy coming in from the heavens to the earth.

Scientifically, the measurable part of this energy is called *cosmic rays*, or energy from the cosmos. Cosmic rays consist of *atomic nuclei* (atoms stripped of their electrons) that travel at nearly the speed of light. Collectively, they are referred to as *primary radiation*. As they spiral inward, cosmic rays interact with the earth's atmosphere, producing what is called *secondary radiation*. An estimated 600 rays pass through the human body every minute.

Although a certain percentage of cosmic rays originate from beyond the galaxy, the majority is generated relatively nearby. The sun emits energy at practically all wavelengths. This electromagnetic energy ranges from long radio waves to the shorter microwaves and infrared, light, ultraviolet, and X-rays. We sense the ultraviolet rays as heat, and see the light waves. Instruments are needed to detect the other forms of radiation.

Another source of energy on earth is the *Van Allen Belt*. It is a huge zone of radiation surrounding the planet, consisting of charged particles captured by the earth's magnetic field. These particles reach the planet's surface mainly at the north and south magnetic poles.

Actually, cosmic radiation represents only the measurable portion of the total energy, collectively called Heaven's force, that we receive. A far greater amount, originating beyond our galaxy, remains undetectable.

Moving on its course from the periphery to the center, Heaven's force reaches its final destination—from our perspective—at the center or core of the earth. Having reached its most condensed state, there is only one direction left to go. Heaven's force begins to reverse direction, moving outward and upward in an expanding motion from the center back toward the periphery. This mirrors the macrobiotic principle that, at their extreme point, all things begin to change into their opposite and complementary tendency.

This opposite force travels on a course to the earth's surface, up through the atmosphere, out into the solar system, and on to the farthest reaches of the universe. This motion or tendency, called yin, is also referred to as Earth's force because of its origin. Its effect is expansion, diffusion, and differentiation. A small segment of Earth's force can be measured in the form of radioactive energy generated by such elements as potassium 40, uranium 238, and thorium 232. From the macrobiotic view, these elements, having reached the extreme point of contraction, represent matter's return to vibration or energy.

On the surface of the earth, the upward growth of the plant kingdom is an example of the influence of Earth's force. (The downward growth of a plant's roots is influenced more by Heaven's force, a reflection of the macrobiotic principle that yin and yang exists in all things, although never in equal proportions.) The effect of Earth's force is also reflected in the fact that Heaven's force, in this case represented by the detectable cosmic rays, enters primarily at the north and south poles (Figure 3). It is less energetic at the equator, where it is deflected by the active upward and expanding energies Earth's force.

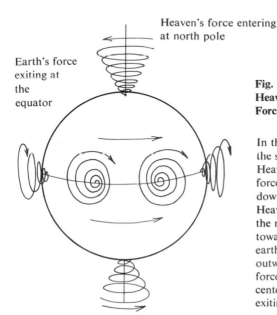

Heaven's force entering at north pole

Earth's force exiting at the equator

Fig. 3 Dynamics of Heaven's and Earth's Forces

In this drawings we see the spirallic energies of Heaven's and Earth's forces. The contracting, downward energy of Heaven's force enters at the north pole and moves toward the center of the earth. The expanding, outward energy of Earth's force is coming from the center of the earth and exiting around the equator.

Fig. 4

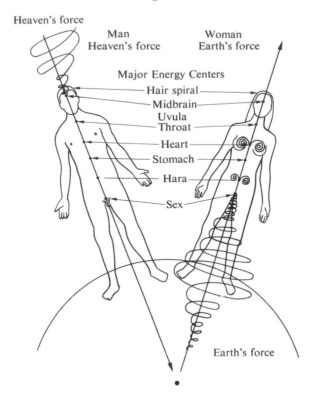

This diagram shows how Heaven's and Earth's forces enter our bodies and pass through them creating a central energy channel. Along these channels are 7 major energy centers from which the forces of Heaven and Earth are distributed throughout the whole body.

Yin and yang, or Heaven's and Earth's force, are the primary forces in the universe (Figure 4). They are the source of all phenomenon, on every level of existence—physical, mental, and spiritual. The interaction of these two forces creates the energy or vibrations that the science of physics tells us is the basis of the material world. They are the source from which all things come, are animated, and return to.

One need not be a scientist to realize that everything is in motion. Day changes into night, summer to winter, childhood to adulthood. There is a pattern, an order to this change. Opposites attract each other to create a balanced or harmonious state. Likes repel each other to maintain this harmony. One tendency changes into its opposite, and then begins to move back to its original state. These cycles appear universally, although their time scale may be too long or too short for us to notice. The obvious patterns of the 24-hour daily cycle, the 28-day lunar cycle, and the 12-month yearly cycle are examples in miniature of the rise and fall of civilizations, and the birth and death of the stars, galaxies, and universes.

The influence of these two primary tendencies appears in various regional climatic and geographical conditions. More northern regions, where cold weather predominates, tend to have less developed plant growth, variety, and color. Areas where warmer weather predominates tend to have larger plant growth, variety, and color. These are reflections of the respective influence of Heaven's and Earth's force. Such geographical features as mountains, exhibit more of the upward tendency of Earth's force, whereas plains and valleys show the effect of Heaven's force.

Creating a view of ourselves, our world, our universe, our origins and destiny is called *cosmology*. Macrobiotic cosmology, with its use of the Unifying Principles of yin and yang, provides the keys to the structure and order of the universe. With these principles, a comprehensive and holistic understanding can be obtained of the nature of any topic we wish to examine. This is as true for governmental policies and economic cycles as it is for diet and healing. The focus of this book is on the application of the macrobiotic principles to the problems of infertility and reproductive disorders. A variety of excellent books are now available, several describing the macrobiotic principles in detail, others explaining their application to particular topics. Readers are referred to the bibliography for a list.

The Human Constitution

Having examined the principles that govern the universe, we can now apply the concept of yin and yang, or Earth's and Heaven's force, to the subject of the human body. Like all other things in creation, the human body is formed and animated by the interaction of these two opposite and complementary forces. All bodily movement, from locomotion to the beating of the heart, is the result of the rhythmic contraction and expansion of various spirals.

Heaven's force enters the human body from above in the region of the hair spiral on the top of the head—our north magnetic pole. From there, it moves downward through the body in a contracting spiralic motion. Earth's force enters the body from below, through the feet, and the genital area—our south magnetic pole. From here, it moves upward through the body in an expanding spiralic motion.

These forces run through the depths of the body, creating a channel of electromagnetic energy referred to as the *Primary Channel*.

These complementary forces, moving in opposite directions along the Primary Channel, create five major energy centers in the body. Together with the two entrance points, this produces seven major areas of active energy charge in the body. These include:

1.   The area around the hair spiral at the top and back part of the head. This center governs higher consciousness, and is the source of universal inspiration and understanding.

2.   The inmost region of the brain, the midbrain. From here energy charges are distributed to the billions of brain cells, stimulating chemical and biological functions such as hormone production in the hypothalamus and pituitary glands. This center is the source of consciousness, wisdom, and spirituality.

3.   The throat region, towards the root of the tongue. The energy charge in this area activates the rhythm of respiration, the secretion of saliva, the operation of the thyroid and parathyroid glands, and the voice. This center governs speech, expression, and harmony with the atmosphere.

4.   The heart region. At this center the energies of Heaven and Earth are most evenly balanced. They activate the rhythmic beating of the heart and the movement of the circulatory system—Earth's force influences the expansion of the heart and the outward movement of blood, while Heaven's force stimulates the heart's contraction, and the blood's inward movement. This energy center governs social harmony and love.

5.   The stomach region. From this center, energy charges the central organs—liver, gall bladder, spleen, pancreas, stomach, and kidneys. This center controls reason and intellect, and coordinates physical and mental activities.

6.   The lower abdomonial region, below the navel. Energy in this center charges the small and large intestine, the bladder, and the sexual organs. In woman, this center is located deep within the uterus where implantation and fetal development occur. Energy from this center controls digestion and absorption. This center governs our physical life-force, and the power and stability of both physical and mental activity.

7.   The genital area. From this center, the reproductive organs and the eliminatory system are activated. This center governs reproductive energy, and our ability to adapt to our surroundings.

From these energy centers, channels of energy, called *meridians* in Oriental medicine, flow. These channels branch out into increasingly smaller streams that nourish every cell in the body. At various locations along the meridians are points, called *tsubo*, where energy exists in various states. These points can be used to determine the degree of health of their related organs and functions. Long before obvious symptoms become apparent, irregularities along the meridian lines and on the tsubo points, such as swolleness, hardness, discoloration, and so on, indicate that imbalances are developing.

Without this comprehensive view, we would have only a limited perception of relationships and interactions within the human body. Our explanations of the structure and functions of organs and systems would consequently be general at best. And our attempts at treatment when problems develop would necessarily be symptomatic.

The different biological, mental, and emotional characteristics found in men and women are the result of the varying degree of influence of Heaven's and Earth's force. Obviously, both sexes are created and activated by a combination of these two forces. Nothing is totally yin or yang. Yet the two sexes differ because of the primary energetic influence they receive. Man reflects more the influence of Heaven's force—wider shoulders, downward and external sexual organs, longer form. Women reflect more the influence of Earth's force—wider hips, upward and internal sexual organs, and a less elongated form. These differences, showing the influence of opposite energies, are the basis for the strong attraction and interaction between the sexes. As mentioned earlier, opposites attracts to achieve balance.

The state of our health is determined by how well the forces of Heaven and Earth flow through our body. Traditional healing arts like acupuncture, massage, and herbal medicine, aim at harmonizing energy that has become either excessive or deficient. The biggest influence on the quality of our energy flow is our way of life, and in particular, our way of eating.

If one eats in accordance with the principles of nature, yin and yang, these energies flow smoothly and generate a strong charge of health. If there are blockages or weaknesses in our body, caused by a diet high in animal foods, simple sugars, and chemicals, for instance, these energies are diminished and our health declines. Over time, the function of organs and systems is affected, and ultimately degeneration begins.

Heaven's and Earth's force, internal energy flow, daily food and drink, emotions, the powers of the mind, spiritual consciousness: an intimate relationship runs through all of these factors—each affects and is affected by the others. Our freedom as human beings lies in our ability to influence each of these by our daily way of life.

Now, with our broad understanding, we are ready to apply the Unifying Principle to the male and female reproductive system.

The Human Reproductive System

As we have seen, Heaven's downward-moving energy creates and energizes the male reproductive system and the characteristics associated with the male sex. Thus, a male's primary reproductive organs (Figure 5) are outside and below the body cavity.

The male reproductive organs descend include: 1) The *penis*; 2) the *testes*; 3) the *scrotum*, the sac which contains the testes; 4) glands, such as the *prostate*, which aid in the formation of seminal fluid used to transport sperm; and 5) a system of tubes for transporting sperm, including the *epididymis* and *seminal ducts* (also called the *vas deferens*).

Fig. 5   The Basic Anatomy of the Male Reproductive System

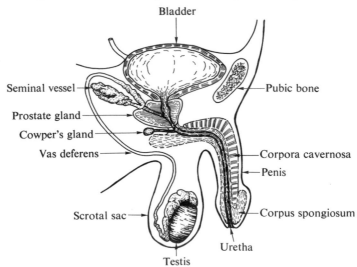

The testes serve two basic functions: They produce *spermatoza*, or sperm, and they produce the male hormones, including *testosterone*, which influences the secondary sexual characteristics which develop at puberty. The inner part of the testicle is divided into chambers, or *lobules*. Each lobule contains tightly wound tubes called *seminiferous tubules*. The cells lining these tubules produce millions of sperm daily. The new sperm are then transported to the epididymis, where they reach maturity. Mature sperm is composed of a head, body, and tail. The head portion contains the genetic material from 23 chromosomes.

In comparison to males, Earth's more expansive energy produces the female reproductive system and many of the qualities associated with the female sex. The female reproductive system (Figure 6) includes: External Sexual Organs: 1) the *labia majora* and *labia minor* (outer and inner lips)—the two folds of soft skin which surround the vagina; 2) the *clitoris*, the small erectile organ which becomes filled with blood during sexual activity. Internal Sexual Organs: 1) the *vagina*, a muscular tube extending upwards and backwards from the vulva; 2) the *cervix*, or narrow neck of the uterus (the lowest portion of the uterus that extends down into the vagina); 3) the *uterus*, a hollow pearshaped organ that lies in the center of the lower abdomen; 4) the *oviducts* or *Fallopian tubes*—paired tubes, about five inches long, extending from the top of the uterus to the ovaries; 5) the *ovaries*, the primary organs of reproduction, located on either side of the uterus.

Fig. 6   The Basic Anatomy of the Female Reproductive System

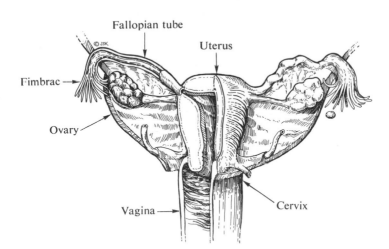

The two basic functions of the ovaries are the production of *ova* (egg cells) and the secretion of the hormones *estrogen* and *progesterone*. The ovarian hormones create feminine bodily and sexual characteristics and play a primary role in the monthly menstrual cycle. The process of egg maturation in the ovary is complementary to sperm development. Males produce millions of sperm in a process of diffusion. Females usually produce just one mature egg in each monthly cycle in a process of condensation.

At birth, the outer layer of each ovary, the *cortex*, contains up to 400,000 immature *primary ovarian follicles*. Each follicle is a spirally formed mass of cells at the center of which lies an ovum, or egg cell. At the start of each menstrual cycle, several follicles begin to mature. Normally, however, only one reaches maturity in each cycle while the others degenerate.

As a follicle matures, it follows a spirallic path inside the ovary, absorbing fluid and swelling into a sac-like structure called the *Graafian follicle*. About ten days from the start of its development, the mature follicle bursts and releases its ovum. This ovum enters the finger-like end of the Fallopian tube, called the *fibrium*. The discharge of the mature ovum is known as *ovulation*, and it occurs about once every twenty-eight days.

Once ovulation has taken place, the ruptured follicle undergoes a transformation, taking the form of a solid, yellow mass of cells called the *corpus luteum* or yellow body. If the ovum is not fertilized, the corpus luteum will grow for twelve to fourteen days, and then degenerate. If conception occurs, the corpus luteum will continue to grow and secrete hormones for about twelve weeks, then the placental hormones take over the support of the pregnancy.

The Menstrual Cycle ───────────────────────

The duration of the menstrual cycle can vary greatly due to individual differences in constitution, lifestyle, and health condition. Generally, the menstrual cycle is about twenty-eight days, a period corresponding to the lunar month. During the menstrual cycle there is an alternating secretion of hormones in the female body (Figure 7).

The pituitary gland, located under the center of the brain, secretes

Fig. 7   The Alternating Order and the Downward and Upward Movement of Female Sexual Hormones During the Menstrual Cycle

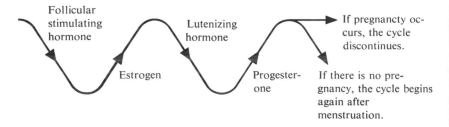

Follicular stimulating hormone

Lutenizing hormone

If pregnancty occurs, the cycle discontinues.

Estrogen

Progesterone

If there is no pregnancy, the cycle begins again after menstruation.

Follicular stimulating hormone (FSH) and Luteinizing hormone (LH). In the ovary, the Grafian follicle secretes estrogen and the corpus luteum secretes progesterone. This hormonal cycle reflects the complementary/antagonistic nature of the forces of Heaven and Earth.

With menstrual discharge, the pituitary gland begins secreting FSH. This hormone moves down into the body through the circulatory system in a process influenced by the downward energy of Heaven's force. Rising levels of FSH stimulate the production of estrogen by the Graafian follicle in the ovary. Estrogen, reflecting the influence of the more expansive, upward-moving energy of Earth's force, complements FSH.

Two things happen as estrogen levels rise: 1) the production of FSH gradually decreases; and 2) the pituitary gland begins to secrete the complementary hormone, LH, a product of Heaven's force. This hormone stimulates final maturation of the egg and then ovulation, at which point the egg leaves the ovary and enters the Fallopian tube.

As a balancing response, progesterone is then secreted by the corpus luteum. This hormone, influenced more by Earth's force, further stimulates the growth of the uterine lining in preparation for the fertilized egg. As progesterone levels increase, the production of LH decreases. If fertilization does not occur, the egg will degenerate and be discharged along with the built-up lining of the uterus.

This alternating increase and decrease of various hormones is a clear example of the complementary nature of Heaven's and Earth's forces. It also reveals our connection to broader environmental influences. This alternating cycle is depicted in Figure 7.

Fig. 8

The menstrual cycle can be divided into two phases. From menstruation to ovulation, biological processes are activated more by Heaven's force. From ovulation to menstruation, biological processes are activated more by Earth's force.

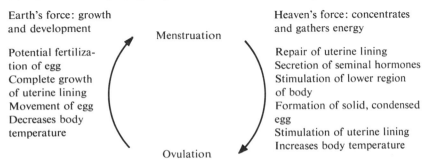

The influence of these hormones overlaps. That is to say, one does not begin and the other end immediately. This is a reflection of the macrobiotic principle that large yin attracts small yin, and large yang attracts small yang. According to the principles of change, at its extreme point, a thing will start to change into its opposite. This is a gradual rather than sudden change. We see this reflected in the progression of the seasons—summer does not abruptly turn into winter. The change is gradual, and consists of the transitional period of autumn.

The twenty-eight day (approximate) menstrual cycle also reflects the order of the universe. Dividing the cycle in half, the first part, from menstruation to ovulation, is influenced more by the contracting, downward force of Heaven. The second half, from ovulation to menstruation, is influenced more by the expanding, upward influence of Earth's force. Of course, within each half, various aspects of Heaven's and Earth's force exist—nothing is completely yin or completely yang.

The Evolution of Reproduction

Reproduction involves the bringing together of an egg cell and a sperm cell to create a new life. For most of the animal kingdom this is the basic biological process for the continuation of the species. However, the sexual act that accomplishes this combination is not the same for all creatures. There are interesting differences which reveal the endless combinations of the antgonistic/complementary nature of the universe.

For example, a general division can be made between aquatic and land creatures. In a water environment, the female releases a large number of eggs which tend to sink in the water. The male also releases large numbers of sperm which then either swim or are carried by currents to the egg. This type of fertilization is *external*, with the ocean, sea, lake, or river providing the liquid medium through which the egg and sperm travel.

Land animals, living in the opposite, or air world, lack this external environment for egg and sperm to move through. Their method of fertilization is consequently also opposite to water animals. They employ *internal* fertilization, in which the male and female physically join or unite, with the union of the egg and sperm occurring inside the female's body. In this case, sperm cells are provided a liquid environment through which to move to the egg by the female reproductive tract. We can see that a darker, cooler, water environment produces one type of fertilization, and its opposite, a brighter, warmer, land environment produces a complementary form of fertilization.

Internal fertilization reflects the evolution of accessory sexual organs used in transferring sperm from the male to the female in the

Fig. 9

During biological evolution, the positions of the spine changed from a more
horizontal position in lower creatures to an increasingly more vertical position
in higher creatures. Humans have a vertical spine. This evolution in spinal position
is correlated to changes in sexual development. Human sexual development is the
most advanced result of this evolution.

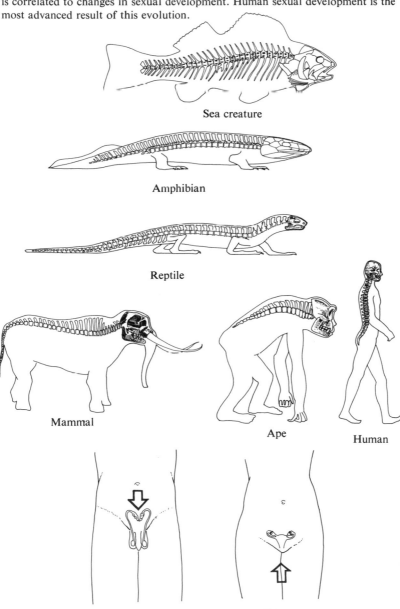

Sea creature

Amphibian

Reptile

Mammal

Ape

Human

Man

Woman

process of sexual union. Amphibians are next in the evolutionary line, following species that survive only in water. Although amphibians can live both on land and in water, their method of fertilization is external. To reproduce, they return to the water or at least to a very moist area. Females lay their eggs in this liquid environment for the male to fertilize.

Next on the evolutionary ladder is reptiles. This class includes snakes, lizards, birds, dinosaurs, and so on. Reptiles employ internal fertilization for reproduction. Following fertilization, the female deposits the eggs outside her body. Reptile eggs have a hard shell enclosing a liquid environment, call the *amnion*, in which the embryo is nourished and develops. This liquid environment is the internalization of the external water environment that lower creatures utilize in their reproduction.

Mammals, the next stage of animal evolution, also utilize internal fertilization. In addition, there is a further sophistication in the reproduction process. In mammals, there is no shell around the fertilized egg. Instead, the fertilized ovum is implanted in the newly evolved female organ, the uterus. The uterus replaces the shell of the egg found in lower animals. The growing embryo develops in a liquid environment called *amniotic fluid*, inside the mother's body.

In mammals, there is a direct link between the mother and the nourishment of the embryo—the baby is nourished from the mother's blood stream. In the placenta, the blood vessels of the embryo and the mother lie close together, but they are not joined, and there is no mixing of maternal and fetal blood. Exchange takes place by diffusion between the two. Nutritive substances and oxygen move from the mother to the embryo, and urinary wastes and carbon dioxide move from the embryo to the mother.

This fact is of great significance. The mother's blood, which is created by the food she eats, nourishes, and in a very real sense, becomes the baby. This process is extended as mammals, unlike lesser evolved creatures, continue to nourish their offspring after birth through the process of breastfeeding.

Human beings, the most highly evolved of all creatures, possess all these abilities, plus a system of single mating—one male to one female. Because we are not tied to a mating season, we also have more control over our reproduction. In addition, humans have a complex structure for the development of the nonphysical aspects of the offspring—the family and the various social and cultural institutions built upon it.

By far, our greatest freedom is the ability to choose our daily food, thus directly affecting the quality of our reproductive cells. This freedom takes on special significance for females, as they exercise their food choices during pregnancy and the period of breastfeeding. After a child is weaned, the mother continues to exert a strong influence on his or her well-being through her cooking.

Evolution of the Reproductive System ─────────

The location, size, and shape of the human reproductive system mirrors the influence of Heaven and Earth upon the body during the course of evolution. (Refer to Figure.—) This can be clearly seen in the changing position of the spine—developing from a more horizontal position in lower creatures to a vertical one in human beings.

In lower aquatic animals, the spine is horizontal in relation to the earth. Amphibians have a more detached, mobile head and neck structure. They can move their heads without having to move their whole spine as a unit. In reptiles, the head and neck is further raised and is capable of more individualized movement. The head and neck of mammals can be raised and lowered, and turned in various directions.

Apes represent a major transition to two-legged, almost upright posture, with the spine in a more vertical position. This posture permitts a much stronger up and down flow of Heaven's and Earth's force. Humans have a fully erect posture with the spine on a vertical axis in relationship with the earth. This spinal position permits a very strong charge and interaction of Heaven's and Earth's force throughout the body.

As this process of spinal development was unfolding, a complementary change was going on in the lower part of the body; the sexual organs and reproductive system were becoming more complex. One obvious refinement was the development of accessory sexual organs that permitted a joining of the male and female during sexual intercourse. The human reproductive system is a direct outcome of the energetic charge of Heaven's and Earth's force made possible by our upright posture. The complementary relationship between the male and female reproductive system is a reflection of the influence of these two forces. This is illustrated in Figure —.

The following summary illustrates the patterns of change that occurred during the evolution of the reproductive system.

1. Decreasing number of eggs secreted. Starting with huge numbers, there is a gradual reduction in the numbers of eggs produced, until, in humans, generally only one egg is secreted per ovulation.

2. Decreasing number of conceptions. In humans only one egg is fertilized as a general rule.

3. Single birth. Throughout the evolutionary chain, the number of births decline until, in humans, there is generally just a single birth per pregnancy.

4. Increasing cellular division resulting in the specialization of cell-groups to produce organs. These organs represent the internalization of the external environment. They provide increasing amounts of freedom to move through one's environment. Examples in the human reproductive system include: Females, amniotic fluid, and the uterus; Males, semen, and the prostate gland and the seminal vessels.

5. Closer link between mother and offspring. The human baby is nourished by the mother's blood, then by her breast milk, and finally by her cooking.

6. Flexible adaptation of food. Humans are free to eat up and down the evolutionary scale, and have the additional ability to alter the influence of their food through cooking.

The location of the human reproductive system in the lower part of the body is complementary/antagonistic to the plant kingdom as a whole. The reproductive organs of plants are located at the top or tip of the plant. Flowers can contain both male and female organs, called the *stamen* and *pistil*. In plants, fertilization takes place at the top, whereas in human beings it takes place in the lower portion of the body. It is also in these respective areas that a special cellular process, called *meiosis*, takes place. The end product of meiosis, for both male and female, is the creation of a cell that contains one-half the chromosomes that a normal cell contains. For example, human cells contain 46 chromosomes but reproductive cells contain half that number, or 23. When male and female cells unite, each carrying 23 chromosomes, the resulting creation of new life contains the 46 chromosomes that all humans have.

Carrying our comparison further, we see the overall complementary/ antagonistic relationship between plants and humans. The root of the plant correlates with the head region of a human, specifically the brain. A root absorbs nourishment from the soil, whereas the brain receives nourishment, in the form of Heaven's force, from the universe. The plant root takes in more material nourishment, while the brain receives a more refined energy.

A plant's stems and branches, which circulate nourishment up and out throughout its body, correlates to the human nervous system, with its numerous branches that distribute Heaven's force down and in throughout the body.

Plants, with their characteristic upward and outward orientation, reflect the influence of Earth's force. Humans, with their more downward and complex internal development, reflect the influence of Heaven's force. Plants feed the human material body, providing nourishment and energy, and creating health. This provides a sound basis for the brain and nervous system to attract increased energy from Heaven's force.

This broad relationship between the plant and animal kingdom is given to clarify the correlation and the dependence of human and animal life upon the plant world. The plant kingdom is the source of our well-being. Recognizing this relationship, and making use of it in our daily life, including our way of eating, helps ensure our development as human beings.

Sexual Intercourse

The attraction between a man and a woman is the never ending attraction between universal opposites seeking to achieve harmony. Next to eating, the sexual act is the strongest impulse that we experience. Eating is the primary means we use to make balance with our environment. If we do not eat, we cease to exist. Without sexual activity, it is not our individual survival that is at risk, but that of our genes.

During sexual intercourse there is a tremendous surge of energies in the bodies of a man and woman, representing the union of Heaven's and Earth's force. This energy is in the form of heat (increased body metabolism and temperature), increased system and organ activity, and an exchange of energy and biological material resulting in the potential fusion of egg and sperm cell.

Strong attraction between a couple is based on the health of the individuals. Each must be vital and strongly charged with their dominant force. Initial sexual excitement is produced by sight, touch, sound, smell, taste, and thought or image. This includes the full scope of our sensory system and our brain and nervous system. In the man there is a surge of blood to the penis that results in an erection. In a woman there is a slight enlargement in the breasts and congestion of the clitoris and labia with added vaginal secretions. When the penis is inserted into the vagina there can be a prolonged period of intense enjoyment leading up to orgasm. Orgasm occurs in the male with a series of very fast contractions of the muscles surrounding the male urethra, that produces ejaculation of the semen. In the female, orgasm occurs as the upper part of the vagina begins to rapidly contract and expand. This action serves to draw the sperm deeper into her body. This is a simplified physiological explanation of sexual intercourse. But there is another approach to understanding sexuality.

Representing different poles of energy, man (Heaven's force) and woman (Earth's force) are naturally attracted to each other to create balance between and within themselves. During sexual intercourse, the man's positively charged, and the woman's negatively charge energy poles—the penis and vagina—are connected. A strong charge starts to build, and its frequency is increased by the the wave-like motion of the couple. As the frequency increases, the charge runs in stronger and stronger waves along the couples' Primary Channel. Rising bodily temperatures increase conductivity. Gradually, a very high voltage is generated. At its peak, or climax, a spark passes through the couple as their opposite energies neutralize each other. Temporarily the partners are balanced with their environment and with the universe. Later, their respective energies will build again, and attraction for the opposite sex will once more be felt.

The number of sperm in an ejaculation can vary greatly. The average is around 300 to 350 million. As the sperm swim upward through the vagina, their numbers decrease. Enzymes dissolve cervical mucus permitting entry of about one million sperm to the uterus. Uterine contractions pull the swimming sperm up to the Fallopian tubes. But here only about one thousand enter. About half enter the Fallopian tube which does not contain a egg and perish. About one hundred sperm reach the ovum (if there is one), but only one fertilizes it. The decreasing number of sperm as they move upward towards the egg represents the evolution of the reproductive system. In lower creatures, huge numbers of eggs are fertilized, but as evolution progressed, this number decreased until, in humans, usually only one egg and one sperm unite.

At the moment of conception, the sperm's head, containing the nuclear material of 23 chromosomes, penetrates the ovum. These combine with the 23 chromosomes of the ovum to form a cell of 46 chromosomes that will begin to divide into a new human being.

The length of time that sperm can survive in the uterus and Fallopian tubes is not precisely known. It is generally thought that they can live for about 48 hours or possibly longer. The length of time that an egg or ovum can be fertilized is generally shorter, about 24 hours or possibly longer. There is a limited time each month, if ovulation is monthly, that conception can possibly occur.

We have already seen how all parts of the body are connected and interrelated. Any part tells us about the whole and the whole is a reflection of the total functioning of the various parts. How well the kidneys and bladder are functioning, for instance, reveals not only the health of the kidneys and bladder but also the whole body. In addition, the kidneys and bladder are closely related to the healthful operation of the reproductive system.

The kidneys are located in the small of the back. They are small bean-shaped organs on each side of the spine in the general area below the rib cage and above the top of the pelvic bone. A pair of tubes, called *ureters*, run from each kidney down to the bladder, which is centrally located in the reproductive region. In the male, the bladder sits atop the prostate gland. In the female, the bladder is between the pubic bone and curve of the uterus, cervix, and vagina.

The kidneys remove wastes from our blood and pass them down to the bladder in the form of liquid acid. The bladder then swells with this liquid waste and eliminates it through urination. The function of the kidneys is closely connected to the heart. The pumping of the heart creates the necessary pressure to push blood down to the kidneys. The kidneys require the constant pressure that the heart provides in order to function efficiently. If blood pressure drops, the adrenal glands, which rest atop each kidney, secrete *renin*, a hormone that will increase blood pressure.

There is a strong antagonistic/complementary relationship between the heart and the kidneys. The heart supports the working of the kidneys, and if it does not, the kidneys will respond by stimulating the secretion of renin. One-quarter of the blood of every heart beat goes to the kidneys. This blood enters the center of each kidney through the renal artery, and moves towards its periphery.

At the periphery are approximately one million *glomeruli*, which consist of a bunched network of capillaries. This is surrounded by a double-membrane structure called *Bowman's capsule*. It is here, through strong expansion and contraction, that blood is filtered through the walls of the capillaries, and moved back toward the center of the kidney through the *nephron*. During this process, most of the glucose, many of the salts, and most of the water (about 99 percent) is reabsorbed into the body. The waste, in the form of uric acid, flows into the ureter which carries it down to the bladder. In 20 to 30 minutes all of the water in our blood is filtered by the kidneys.

This whole process occurs because of the strong expansion and contraction of the heart, which creates the pressure necessary to move blood down to the kidneys. This strong downward energy is also accompanied by expansion, the movement of blood toward the periphery of the kidneys. An opposite movement then begins with a return toward the center of the kidneys and with the downward movement of waste to the bladder. This results in the expansion of the bladder, which again becomes its opposite, resulting in contraction and urination. This endless cycle of contraction and expansion reflects the energy of Heaven's and Earth's force in our body.

The kidney's function has changed through evolution. Dividing the animal kingdom between aquatic creatures and land creatures, kidney function in aquatic creatures serves to remove waste from the blood. These wastes are excreted into an external liquid environment. With the evolution of creatures to a land or air environment, this basic process of excretion continued. However, living in air represented an opposite environment from the previous liquid one. As a result the kidneys, besides eliminating waste, evolved the new function of reabsorbing water after filtration. This retaining of water was needed to maintain balance between the animal's internal environment and the drier land and air environment.

In males, the channel through which urination occurs is the same channel through which semen travels through the penis. Problems in the bladder, which is physically connected to the kidney, will strongly influence the movement of semen and hence the reproductive system. In females, the urinary system is separated from the reproductive system. The *urethra*, the channel carrying urine from the bladder during urination, leads into the vulva. Although these two are separate, they are in close physical contact and their individual functions exert a strong influence upon one another.

There is a close anatomical relationship between the kidneys and bladder and the reproductive system, and there is also a close energy relationship. We have described the movement of Heaven's and Earth's force through the body. Meridians carry this energy to every part of our body, stimulating, activating, and regulating its various functions. Our organs are part of this system of energy circulation. Each organ is part of a meridian, receiving energy that stimulates it. For example, the bladder, as all our organs do, functions by expanding and contracting. Physically the bladder expands with uric acid from the kidney. The energy that stimulates or triggers urination is conducted by the bladder meridian which runs from the head down through the body along the spine, into the bladder, and then down the back of our legs to the foot. This downward flow of energy channels Heaven's contracting force to the bladder, stimulating its contraction and allowing us to urinate. Energy going to the bladder and the kidneys is also distributed to the reproductive system where it stimulates various related functions. Because this energy relationship is unseen, its influence on the body's physical functions has only currently begun to be explored. Recently, interest has been stimulated by the increasing acceptance of acupuncture in this country.

The basis of the healthful physical and energetic functioning of the reproductive system is linked to the healthful physical and energetic functioning of the kidneys and bladder. This relationship is like the relationship between husband and wife. If there is a problem with one partner there will be a problem with the other in varying degrees.

Conclusion

In this chapter we have looked at the body in terms of yin (Earth's force) and yang (Heaven's force). This understanding has been applied to the male and female reproductive system to see not only its physical characteristics but the energy behind its functioning. We have also examined biological evolution and various changes that have taken place in the male and female reproductive system. With this basis of information we can now focus specifically on the physically related (designated) causes of infertility and reproductive disorders that can lead to infertility.

3. Infertility ▬▬▬▬▬▬▬▬▬▬

We have already seen how the macrobiotic approach to infertility and reproductive disorders aims at eliminating the underlying cause of the problem. In many cases, infertile couples could regain their ability to have children by following macrobiotic dietary and way of life recommendations, with specific modifications for individual circumstances. In this chapter we will discuss the particular problems that are commonly associated with these disorders. It must be remembered, however, that ultimately one's way of life and view of life lead to the circumstances that create such conditions. This idea will be discussed in more detail later in the book.

Problems Associated with Infertility ▬▬▬▬▬▬▬▬

Although all physical problems are reflected in the vitality and health of male and female reproductive functions, certain conditions have a stronger and more direct influence.

1. *Sexually Transmitted Disease (STD):* Sexually Transmitted Disease is a category of illnesses that includes a wide variety of diseases that can be transmitted by sexual contact. Examples of the better-known STDs include *gonorrhea, syphilis, herpes simplex virus 2, chlamydia, trichomoniasis,* and *chancroid.* Each of these can cause severe damage to the reproductive system.

In men, STDs can weaken sperm production, damage the testes and the network of tubes in the sperm transport system, reduce sexual vitality and performance, and in general lead to an all-around low level of resistance.

In women, STDs can be especially damaging to the reproductive tract. They can produce lingering infections, scarring and adhesions throughout the pelvic region—the Fallopian tubes are particularly vulnerable—which can block the movement of the egg and the sperm, thus causing infertility. Chlamydia infection, for example, is considered the most harmful of all pelvic infections. It is the leading cause of female infertility among STDs. It can strike any part of the male or female reproductive tract. In men, chlamydia can cause *urethritis,* which is an inflammation of the urinary passageway. This inflammation can spread to the epididymis, causing swelling and inflammation of the testes, and in turn produce male infertility.

In woman, chlamydia infection can scar the Fallopian tubes. The result can be infertility or *ectopic pregnancy*—in which implantation of the fertilized ovum takes place in the tubes rather than the uterus. Chlamydia is also associated with an increased risk of miscarriage and premature deliveries. Chlamydia infections are estimated to strike at least 4.6 million men and women in the United States each year.

The active stages of STDs are labeled the *virulent state*. Many STDs, however, can still be transmitted during their inactive or *quiescent stage*, when symptoms do not appear. Because many carriers of various STDs are assymptomatic, and perhaps do not realize they have the disease, the spread of STDs is widespread.

Herpes simplex virus 2 (HSV-2), sometimes called *genital herpes*, is perhaps the most well-known of all STDs. According to the Federal Center for Disease Control, between 25 million and 100 million Americans have the virus. Like other members of the herpes family, HSV-2 sets up a lifelong infection that alternates between virulent and quiescent states. Even when herpes is quiescent, it can be transmitted.

Symptoms during the initial infection can include fever, pain and itching in the genital area, genital blisters that become ulcers, and sometimes headache, stiff neck, and shooting pains in the legs.

Just several years ago, words like epidemic and plague were used to describe the increase in the incidence of genital herpes. More accurate would be the word *pandemic*, meaning common or universal. With the advent of AIDS, however, attention has shifted from what is perceived as a nuisance disease to the killer disease.

2. *Tonsillectomy and Adenoidectomy*, respectively surgical removal of the tonsils and the adenoids, were at one time performed almost routinely. Although this is no longer so, many of us have had these glands removed.

The tonsils are an important part of the lymphatic system. In their function as filters for lymph, they localize and neutralize toxins that would otherwise remain in general circulation. When the tonsils are removed, the remaining parts of the lymphatic system must work harder. The adenoids serve a similar function.

The head and trunk of the body have a complementary relationship. The structure and function of the one is mirrored in the other. The adenoids and testes reflect this relationship. Physically and energetically, they balance one another. If the adenoids are removed, the function of the testes will be weakened. In a similar way, the tonsils and ovaries exist in an complementary/antagonistic relationship. Removal of the tonsils will have a direct effect on ovarian function.

3. *The appendix* reflects the dynamic balance found everywhere in the body. Located in the lower, right portion of the abdomen, this compact organ balances the more expanded structure of the large and small intestines. Removal of the appendix leads to a weakening of the lower body, including digestion and elimination, and the functioning of the sexual organs.

4. *The endocrine system* has a direct effect on reproductive functions of both sexes. Glandular disorders can distort the development of the secondary sexual characteristics that emerge at puberty. In males, they also can upset sperm production by influencing male reproductive hormones.

The vital relationship between the endocrine system and the female reproductive cycle has been examined elsewhere in this book. The timing and balance of hormone secretion is crucial to the smooth unfolding of the menstrual cycle. The pituitary, thyroid, adrenal, and sexual hormones all play a synchronized role in this balance. If there is either an excess or deficiency in any of them, the whole system is upset.

Synthetic hormones can be prescribed for both males and females. Although they can provide temporary, symptomatic relief, they are no substitute for the normal functioning of the glands. The quality, quantity, and timing of hormone secretion is geared to individual needs, and in response to the overall condition of the individual. At best, synthetic hormones provide a general approximation of the intricate ebb and flow of the normal hormonal cycle.

The adrenal glands, located atop the kidneys, have an important role in the endrocrine system. They perform many functions including regulating metabolism of nutrients and the functioning of the parasympathetic branch of the autonomic nervous system. The greatest complementary relationship within the endrocrine system exists between the pituitary and adrenal glands. Other endocrine glands can be considered branches of these two.

The pancreas secretes both digestive juices and the complementary/ antagonistic hormones—insulin and *anti-insulin* (glucagon)—which regulate blood-sugar levels. Imbalances in the pancreas can strongly affect vitality and energy levels, including sexual vitality.

Allergies are a response of the body's immune system to external and internal factors. An allergic response can develop in response to excessive or toxic factors. These same factors can disrupt the structure and function of the reproductive system, producing various blockages and growths, and affecting circulation and hormone quality.

5. *Malnutrition* can affect both underweight individuals and those who are overweight. The quantity of food consumed, at least in industrialized countries, is secondary to the types of food eaten and the condition of the digestive organs. The diets of many individuals are nutritionally lacking. In addition, extreme factors in certain foods, simple sugars and animal fats for example, can restrict the assimilation of nutrients. Obviously, this can lead to a chronic lack of vitality, and eventually, to a weakening of all organs and systems. These same factors can produce accumulations of excess within and around the reproductive organs, leading to a variety of disorders, including blockages, tumors, and cysts. Such deposits can also set the stage for damaging infections within the reproductive system.

Due to social pressures to be slim, many women have tried various "diets" which tend to fall in one of two general categories. The first can be called the *starvation diet*, with the goal to lose weight as rapidly as possible. This has obvious dangers, as it deprives the body of nutrition, and leads to many health problems, including general weakening of vitality.

The second type of diet can be called the *miracle diet*. These programs promise wonderous and instantaneous results if some narrow combination of foods is eaten. Again, basic nutritional needs are ignored in the hope of quick weight loss. Both of these categories can damage reproductive abilities.

5. *The condition of the kidneys and bladder* directly influence reproductive functions. A problem in either of these organs will be reflected in the health and vitality of reproductive functions. This includes infections, stones, tumors, and any degenerative disorder of the kidneys or bladder.

6. *The excessive use of alcohol* has a strong body-wide effect. Alcohol has a yin or expansive influence on the body. Males, primarily energized by Heaven's more yang force, can be weakened in a variety of ways by alcohol abuse. This can include lower sperm counts and a weakening of sperm motility, as well as diminished sexual vitality.

Many cultures have traditions that show recognition of this fact. For example, the Romans believed that Vulcan, the blacksmith of the gods, was born lame because his father, Jupiter, was drunk when he begot Vulcan.

Alcohol also has a direct effect on woman's reproductive health. This is especially true during the first half of the menstrual cycle —from menstruation to ovulation—which is influenced by the downward influence of Heaven's force. The dangers of alcohol during pregnancy have been widely publicized.

Many drugs, licit and illicit, are far more extremely yin than alcohol. This includes marijuana, speed, cocaine, heroine, LSD, nitrate inhalants, so on. These and other such substances weaken all bodily functions and systems, including sexual vitality and reproductive abilities.

7. *Psychological imbalances* can also affect the reproductive system. Unfortunately, they are widespread in the United States and other modern societies. As we have seen, the body, mind, and spirit are inseparable; problems affecting one area will show up in the others. Although psychological disorders manifest mentally, they represent a biochemical and energetic imbalance in the body, including the brain and nervous system. Medications to treat such problems often cause their own set of problems.

Male Reproductive Problems

Infertility affects at least 15 percent of the married couples in the United States. In about 90 percent of the cases, a cause can be found. *Male infertility*, defined as the inability to fertilize the ovum, is involved approximately 40 percent of the time. There are several basic ways in which a male's fertility can be affected: 1) problems with semen quality; 2) problems with sperm production—low numbers, poor motility, malformation; and 3) a blockage or other problem that interferes with sperm delivery.

Other factors, however, may be involved: Injury, congenital problems, and infections, especially the mumps after puberty, are examples.

Semen analysis refers to a series of tests on the seminal fluid to examine various factors. If seminal fluid is too thick, sperm may be unable to move through the semen. This may be caused by infection, in which case antibiotics are prescribed. Interestingly, if the semen is naturally *viscous*, or thick, high doses of vitamin C may be recommended. Vitamin C is a more yin substance, and will thus have a diluting effect on the seminal fluid. However, this expansion will be felt body-wide, and in excess it will weaken the testes in general.

The volume of the seminal fluid will also be checked. If it is too low, the transport of sperm will be impaired, thus interfering with fertility. If too high, sperm density is lowered and motility is reduced.

The pH factor of the seminal fluid will next be taken to determine its degree of acidity or alkalinity. On a scale from 1 to 14, 1 is the most acid, 14 is most alkaline, and 7, the pH of water, is neutral. Seminal fluid is generally slightly alkaline, ranging between 7.0 and 8.5.

As mentioned above, sperm production is evaluated by three basic factors: their number, their shape, and their motility or ability to move or swim. It is no secret that sperm counts have been declining in recent decades. A recent study found that average sperm counts were almost 40 percent lower than in 1920. In a study involving college students, 23 percent were found to have sperm counts so low that they were considered sterile.

The situation is clearly described in the following quote from *The Infertility Handbook*, by Joseph Bellina and Josleen Wilson:

> The decline [in sperm counts] was first noticed in the mid-1970s, when fertility clinics in Texas and New Jersey discovered that men coming in for vasectomies—that is, men assumed to be fertile—had sperm counts considerably lower than the standard defined by MacLeod and Gold. A significant number of these newly tested men had counts of 60 million sperm per ejaculate or less.
>   . . . However, most researchers don't believe the dip in sperm concentration is responsibile for the present infertility epidemic. They consider the dip a normal fluctuation. Accordingly, they have adjusted the average 'normal" sperm count downwards. Technically speaking, a man is considered probably fertile today if his sperm count exceeds 60 million sperm per ejaculate, about half the original number established in the 1950s.

There is a general rule of thumb in sperm-count evaluation called the "rule of the 60s." It defines a normal sperm count as 60 percent normal shape, 60 percent motility, and 60 million sperm per ejaculate. There is, however, a large range of variation in the normal range.

Count. The number of sperm in an ejaculation can vary greatly from individual to individual. Generally each milliliter contains about 100 million sperm. As mentioned above, the minimum requirement for normal sperm count is 60 million. A condition known as *subfertility* ensues when sperm counts drop below this point. If sperm numbers go below 5 to 10 million, infertility is assumed.

Shape. The normal structure of the sperm consists of a head, body or middle section, and a tail (Figure 10). It is generally assumed that there are abnormally formed sperm in the ejaculate of all men. As the percentage of deformed or immature sperm increases the like-

Fig. 10

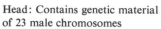

Head: Contains genetic material of 23 male chromosomes

Body: Mitochondria provides energy storage for cell metabolism

Tail: Provides alternate wave motion that propels sperm

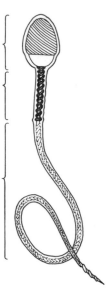

Fig. 11

2 heads

2 heads + 2 tails

Not fully formed

Mitochondria is split in these two sperm.

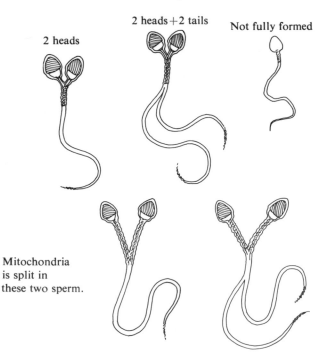

lihood of fertility declines. Examples of deformed sperm can be seen in Figure 11.

Motility.   Sperm motility refers to the degree of vitality or energy of sperm to propel themselves through the female reproductive tract. Sperm motility is judged by the number of sperm swimming and the quality of their movement.

One of the leading causes of male infertility is the condition know as *varicocele*, or varicose vein of the testicle. It is estimated that about 10 percent of all men have a varicocele, and usually it is harmless. It is caused when one or more valves in the vein breaks down causing blood to pool. As the pool of blood increases, the vein begins to swell. This is a varicocele. This pooled blood overheats the testicle's sperm-production centers, and can kill sperm outright. It may also result in immature or deformed sperm, and decreased motility.

After sperm are produced in the testicles, they are pumped through a system of tubes that are joined at intervals by glands that provide seminal fluid. Blockages may develop in these tubes, preventing the ejaculation of sperm. Such blockages are caused by infection, injury, or by an accumulation of fat and protein. The passages through which sperm travel include the epididymis, vas deferens, and ejaculatory ducts (Figure 12).

Fig. 12   Male testis: The basic anatomy of the male testis is shown in this diagram.

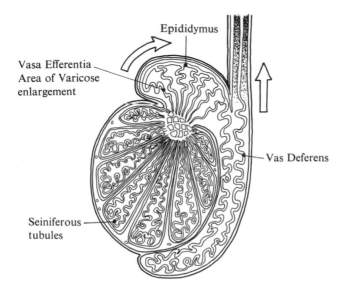

Epididymus

Vasa Efferentia
Area of Varicose
enlargement

Vas Deferens

Seiniferous
tubules

Fig. 13
Various health problems can strike the male reproductive system. In addition, STDS (sexually transmitted diseases) can also damage the whole reproductive tarct.

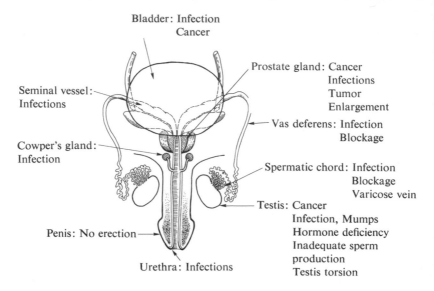

Bladder: Infection
Cancer

Prostate gland: Cancer
Infections
Tumor
Enlargement

Seminal vessel:
Infections

Vas deferens: Infection
Blockage

Cowper's gland:
Infection

Spermatic chord: Infection
Blockage
Varicose vein

Penis: No erection

Testis: Cancer
Infection, Mumps
Hormone deficiency
Inadequate sperm
production
Testis torsion

Urethra: Infections

Female Infertility

Except in the country of India, women everywhere outlive men. In India the rate is lower because women die at an abnormally high rate during pregnancy and childbirth. The country where women live the longest is Japan, where the average lifespan is 80.18 years. Sweden is in second place, with an average lifespan for women of 79.61 years. Women in the United States live an average 78.2 years.

Biologically, women are at the center of the spiral of evolution. They are physiologically more complex than men, a fact reflected in their role as the bearer of new life. Women nourish life before and after birth. In their traditional role as the center of the home, this was extended from physical care to emotional, intellectual, and spiritual nourishment as well. For thousands of years, women were the center of family life, and by extension, the builders of society. Too often, however, this position has been unrecognized and little appreciated.

Unfortunately, the role of woman as mother and homemaker has come under a great deal of criticism in recent years. This is in part due to the shift in modern societies away from an equal partnership of complemental responsibilities between husband and wife. This, in turn, is due to the rapid and pervasive changes in the economic and social makeup of society.

Clearly, there is an antagonistic/complementary relationship between the male and female sex. This includes biological as well as all other aspects of the self. Historically, when this balance between the sexes has shifted, there has been an inevitable reaction to reestablish equilibrium. This process is now going on.

Today, many women are attempting to ignore their innate strengths and abilities and pursuing what has traditionally been a man's role. To a degree, this is understandable. In our rapidly changing world, we are all adjusting to profound shifts in social conditions. As illustrated by decreasing sperm counts, for instance, men are perhaps becoming less masculine.

The danger, however, is that more and more women will abandon, either voluntarily or by economic and social necessity, their complementary role in the male/female equation. As this happens, the biological health of women in particular, and the health of society in general, will be profoundly affected.

The following statistics, published in the September 15 issue of *Parade* magazine, help to bring this point home. The most frequently performed operations as of 1982 in the United States, are listed.

1. Biopsy—the removal of tissue from a living subject for diagnostic purposes.
2. Dilation and Curettage—the expansion and cleaning of the womb for diagnostic or therapeutic purposes.
3. Caesarean section—the operation by which a fetus is taken from the uterus by cutting through the walls of the abdomen.
4. Excision of lesion of skin or tissue.
5. Hysterectomy—the removal of the uterus.
6. Bilateral destruction or occlusion of the Fallopian tubes.
7. Extraction of lens (removal) of a cataract.
8. Repair of inguinal hernia.
9. Oophorectomy and salpingo-oophorectomy—removal of ovaries and Fallopian tubes.
10. Cholecystectomy—removal of the gallbladder.

These statistics reveal that fully half of the surgery performed in the United States involves women exclusively, and more specifically, women's reproductive systems (numbers 2, 3, 5, 6, and 9). This indicates that the biological integrity of women is degenerating rapidly, and this degeneration is particularly pervasive in the reproductive tract. The implications are clear, if not widely acknowledged.

Female Infertility Examined ━━━━━━━━━━━

As mentioned earlier, any health problem will affect reproductive functions and abilities. Following is a discussion of the major medical problems that most often result in female infertility.

1. *Endometriosis.* For women over twenty-five, endometriosis is the leading cause of infertility. Endometriosis occurs when portions of the *endometrium*—the lining of the uterus—break away and start to grow in other areas of the pelvis. This can include the exterior of the uterus, Fallopian tubes, the ovaries, and the surface of the bladder.

This misplaced endometrium menstruates monthly in response to hormones, although it is not discharged. The cycle is growth, bleeding, and regeneration, which can cause scarring, adhesions, and cysts around the uterus, ovaries, and Fallopian tubes. Even in mild cases, this condition can affect fertility by affecting hormonal balance. Symptoms include: 1) severe menstrual pain, 2) deep abdominal discomfort, 3) back pain, and 4) pain during intercourse.

Women in their thirties, who have not given birth, are especially susceptible. If not severe, endometriosis is treated with hormone

Fig. 14

Some of the major health problems that can strike the female reproductive system are shown in this figure. In addition, STDs (sexually transmitted diseases) can damage the whole reproductive tract.

Fallopian tube: Infection
Scaring and adhesion
Narrowing of tube
Twisting
Endometriosis

Uterus: Congenital defects
Cancer
Infections
Tumors, Fibroid (benign or malignant)
Endometriosis

Fimbrae:
Closure

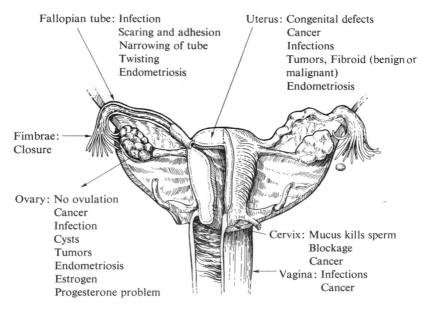

Ovary: No ovulation
Cancer
Infection
Cysts
Tumors
Endometriosis
Estrogen
Progesterone problem

Cervix: Mucus kills sperm
Blockage
Cancer
Vagina: Infections
Cancer

therapy and surgery. If severe, extensive surgery may be required. The symptomatic nature of these procedures is shown in the fact that in many cases, this condition returns within a year of treatment.

2. *Pelvic Inflammatory Disease:* Pelvic Inflammatory Disease (PID) is a widespread condition that can strike throughout the female reproductive system and abdominal area. About one million cases a year are treated in the United States. PID can cause scar tissue and adhesions anywhere in the reproductive tract. Symptoms vary according to the severity of the infection, and can include: 1) vaginal discharge, 2) itching, 3) slight discomfort, 4) painful cramping, and 5) fever.

Causes include sexually transmitted disease, especially gonorrhea and chlamydia, multiple sex partners, abortions, and the use of Intra Uterine Devices (IUD).

3. *Failure to Ovulate:* More than half of all female infertility is due to ovulatory problems. Most often the cause is linked to hormonal disorders that prevent a mature ovum from being released during the menstrual cycle. Erratic menstrual patterns may be the only obvious symptom of this condition. However, a large number of women who are not ovulating still have regular menstrual cycles.

Oral contraceptive pills are the most common cause of this problem. Hormones in the pill take over for the hormones normally produced by the brain-control centers and the ovaries. After going off the pill, about 10 to 15 percent of women experience trouble ovulating. Stress and nutritional imbalance are also factors that can cause ovulation failure and hormonal imbalance.

One of the most common causes of ovulatory problems is a condition called *polycystic ovaries*. Although no cause has been found, it is considered a hormonal problem. In this case, the ovum or egg does not burst out of the Graafian follicle to begin its journey down the Fallopian tube. Instead, the follicle grows into a cyst which clogs the ovary, and interferes with subsequent egg production. A course of drug treatments with "superfertility" drugs is usually recommended.

4. *Fallopian tube blockage.* Blockages of one or both Fallopian tubes is a common problem in female infertility. It may result from pelvic inflammatory disease, endometriosis, or the use of an IUD contraceptive device. Many blockages have no apparent cause.

In general, three things can happen to the Fallopian tube to cause blockage. 1) the *fimbria*, the finger-like end of the Faliopian tube, may scar over, deforming its structure and blocking the upper entrance to the tube, 2) scar tissue can build up around the tubes, effectively tying knots in them, and 3) infection can cause the inner walls of the tubes to stick together, thus causing an obstruction.

5. *Uterine problems.* Although less likely to be involved in infertility, a variety of uterine problems are implicated. These include; 1) developmental or birth defects, in which a segment of the reproductive system is malformed or missing, 2) scarring caused by infection or surgery, or 3) fibroid tumors that interfere with implantion of the embryo.

The most common uterine problem is fibroid tumors. These are usually benign fibrous growths that develop in the uterine wall. This condition affects approximately one women in four in the 30- to 50-age group. Fibroids can interfere with implantation, so that although conception has occurred, the fetus is spontaneously aborted. They may also block the opening from the uterus into the Fallopian tube, thus preventing conception.

6. *Cervical problems.* The cervix is the lowest portion of the uterus. It extends down into the vagina. During the period of ovulation the cervical mucus aids the sperm in the ascent into the uterus. During the rest of the menstrual cycle it prevents the entrance of bacteria. The cervix itself helps to hold the fetus in the uterus during pregnancy. About 10 to 15 percent of female fertility problems are caused by cervical disorders.

Cervical stenosis refers to the condition in which the cervical canal is completely or partially blocked. Polyps, tumors, injury, and scarring are some of the causes. *Hostile cervical mucus* is the condition in which the normally slightly alkaline state of the cervical mucus during ovulation is acidic. This acidic condition either kills or immobilizes the sperm.

Now that we have examined various problems associated with infertility and reproductive disorders, it is time to look at the underlying causes.

4. Diet, Lifestyle, and Reproductive Health ━━━━━━━━

Lifestyle refers to the way we live our life. It consists of the various factors that make up the pattern of our day-to-day existence. To a very large degree, lifestyle is created in response to societal demands. In other words, in order to function in a particular society, we adopt a certain lifestyle. Within this large societal framework, there is quite a bit of flexibility, depending on personal values and goals. Several key factors can be identified that will provide insight into individual lifestyle choices.

1. *The speed or pace of life.*   The pace of life today is fast and getting faster. The rate of change that each of us must come to terms with can be overwhelming. In order to adjust, we set priorities, identifying particular factors as important, and others as marginal or expendable. Too often, one of the first things that suffers is the family experience. This creates a spiral of family disintegration in which family bonds, weakened by lack of shared experience, are loosened, creating in turn less incentive for interaction.

A key factor in the family experience is the sharing of meals. Historically, mealtimes were occasions when family members gathered, discussed problems and experiences, and in general reinforced the feeling of solidarity. Today, family meals are a vanishing phenomenon. Cooking is considered a burden. It is a time-consuming task, which, thanks to modern conveniences, is no longer necessary. Home cooking is taking on the aura of a speciality, a hobby to be pursued perhaps only on weekends. The kitchen is becoming an extension of fast-food restaurants. It is a place were industrially prepared foods are warmed up, often in microwave ovens, and eaten at the individual's convenience. Several decades ago "T.V. dinners" were introduced. At first housewives were skeptical, now prepackaged meals are a basic part of modern life.

Because of schedule conflicts, when family members do eat at home, they are likely to do so alone. The unifying experience of eating together has become a casualty of the pace of modern life. It is important to remember, however, that although this trend is now pervasive, it is a matter of individual choice and priorities.

2. *Personal evaluation or self-reflection.*   Personal evaluation refers

to the habit of examining both the things that happen to us in daily life and the way we react to them. Self-reflection is an attempt to see how our behavior and attitudes are responsible for our circumstances, and an invaluable tool for continual personal growth. It is an efficient means of recognizing the dynamics of cause and effect in our lives. In the words of one time-management expert, "When we fail to relate our todays to our tomorrows [and our yesterdays to our todays] we find ourselves starting from scratch each day. We are left with the grim realization that our wheels are spinning but we aren't going anywhere." Keeping a diary represents one method of self-reflection.

It seems that the only time people self-reflect is when they are faced with some overwhelming difficulty. Serious illness is a good example. This is why macrobiotics teaches that difficulties are beneficial—they make us stop and think. People are sometimes surprised, when listening to accounts of individuals who have reversed a serious problem through the macrobiotic way of life, to hear the individual express gratitude for his or her difficulty. The explanation is that the problem was the motivator that prompted that particular individual to look at his or her way of life, and perhaps for the first time see how unsatisfying and empty it was.

Self-reflection is an important part of health-maintenance and prevention. And, it is essential for anyone wishing to alter personal problems. Daily self-reflection alerts us to small problems that, if unchanged, could turn into serious ones. More importantly, it provides the insights necessary for personal growth throughout our life.

3. *The search for comfort and convenience.* Life in modern society seems to be a relentless search for comfort and convenience. At one time this was understandable. The onset of the Industrial Revolution brought about staggering changes in society. With the destruction of traditional lifestyles, the expectations of many individuals were bleak, and daily life was a constant struggle. In response, our grandparents and great-grandparents set out to improve life for their sons and daughters. Great personal sacrifices were made to foster the prospects of the next generation. The life stories of many prominent individuals illustrates this.

In an incredibly short time, the dreams of our forebears were realized. They were successful beyond their imagining—too successful. Instead of using the convenience of modern life as a means for personal growth, it has become its own end. The amount of disposable income and free time available to all but those on the lowest socio-economic levels surpasses anything know in history. Most of us live in more physical luxury than kings and queens of old. And yet what do we do with this treasure. Too often, we spend our time watching television, and spend our money on more and bigger conveniences.

Physicially, we treat ourselves as invalids, and intellectually we stagnate. Spirituality is the area that we sacrifice in the name of practicality.

4. *Mass Culture.* The benefits of mass production cannot be denied. But like our search for convenience, we have gone too far—we have sacrificed quality for quantity, and extended the concept of mass production to every area of life. From education to medicine, the emphasis is on short-term goals and appearances, rather than enduring quality. Educators point with pride at the high percentage of high-school graduates in this country. No matter that many lack basic reading, writing, and mathematical skills.

Modern society is dominated by the ethics of consumption at the expense of production, and "instant gratification" at the expense of planning and working towards goals.

In no area is this more easily seen, and the results suicidally contradictory, than in the mass production of food. We now have a food industry and like all industries, its primary goal, perhaps its only goal, is profit. Food has been reduced to an economic unit. The cheaper it is produced, the greater the profit. Decisions are made by accountants. Anything that lowers the unit-production cost is adopted.

From this point of view, farming is related to an economic exercise. Thus it makes sense to use chemical fertilizers to make food plants large, to apply chemical pesticides to maximize yields, and to employ farming practices that cut costs as they destroy the soil. Within the last ten years there has been a growing public awareness of the true costs of these trends. We are seeing that these short-term goals, limited to considerations of profit and loss, are inefficient and ultimately ruinous.

Macrobiotics has been a leader in this field. By explaining the long-term as well as the short-term effects and costs, a new accountability is emerging. Stressing fresh, whole, locally grown foods in preference to processed and chemicalized products, a new common sense is emerging. Reasoning from the total spectrum of human considerations—taste, nutrition, health, family and social economy, ecology, and so on—macrobiotic education has brought home the true impact of our food choices.

There is a complemental/antagonistic relationship between individuals and social institutions. Recognizing the practicality of the macrobiotic approach to food production and diet, individuals and families enjoy the freedom and flexibility to alter their consumption patterns. Social institutions, being more insulated from economic, health, and ecological realities, and having less flexibility, require more time to change their policies. Even in the face of overwhelming evidence, other considerations may hold sway. Factors such as the influence of special-interest groups, a lack of understanding on how to implement new policy, or a reluctance to upset the status quo, often are the determining factors.

Ironically, social change in the modern world often happens from the bottom up. Personal habits change, move through the social and economic ladder, and when they have become an established, though as yet unsanctioned way of life, they begin to attract recognition by governing boards of various institutions. The message is clear: individuals and families must take responsibility for their well-being.

The Importance of Food

Since nothing can come out of a human being except from what goes into him, one must assume a close connection between food and fertility. In general, the more generous the diet, the higher the fertility, the more meager the diet, the lower the fertility. However, it is not simply a matter of gross quantity of food. Wealthier people eat better than poor people but they have fewer children.

The above quote, from *Diet and Disease* by Cheraskin, Ringsdorf, and Clark, exhibits a basic common sense that we can all understand. We eat, therefore we are. What we are is the result of what we eat. There is now clinical evidence to suggest the crucial link between diet and reproductive health. Admittedly, this evidence is still incomplete. Even so, although definitive conclusions cannot be scientifically made because of the lack of studies, there is a general consensus about the importance of diet in the functioning of our reproductive systems.

In the summary to their chapter on infertility, the authors listed above, concluded, "Although much remains to be learned about the role of diet in gonadal functions, food does seem to be an important determinant of fertility in both sexes. . . . there has been little effort to evaluate the effect of truly comprehensive dietotherapy under well-controlled conditions . . . such studies seem warranted and perhaps imperative."

From another point of view, Ashley Montagu writes in *Life Before Birth*, "A mother's nutrition is the most important single environmental influence in the life of her unborn child, and it is by means of the food that she eats that a mother can have the most profound and lasting effect on her child's development." What could also be mentioned here is that nutrition is also the single most important environmental influence upon the health of the mother herself. In order to nourish a child she must first have the health and strength to be able to conceive. (This includes the male and the quality of his sperm. If either partner has a severe problem they will not be able to create strong, healthy egg cells and sperm cells.)

Dr. Genevieve Stearns, a University of Iowa nutritionist, has written of the importance of prenatal nutrition. "The best provision for well-being in any period of life is to arrive at that point in good nutritional and physical status. The well-born infant is sturdier throughout infancy than the baby poorly born; the sturdy infant has stores to give impetus to growth in pre-school years. The child who is in excellent nutrition will have stores to be drawn upon during the rapid growth of puberty. The well-nourished mother can nourish her fetus well, therefore the best insurance for a healthy infant is a mother who is healthy and well-nourished throughout her entire life, as well as during the period of pregnancy itself."

In studies on the effect of food upon fertility, the general approach is to isolate one element and analyze its influence by means of deprivation tests. The goal is to determine the effect on the body of the lack of a certain element. This orientation fails to take into account the dynamic interaction of one's overall diet. Subsequent recommendations based on specific food elements leave us to puzzle over ways to incorporate them into a coherent dietary plan. The chemical structures of specific food elements, whether from natural or synthetic sources, are similar. However, their effects on the human body will differ dramatically.

Many food producers advertise that their products contain added nutrients. They fail to mention that it is their own processing methods that leave food devoid of nutritional value, thus necessitating partial supplementation.

Pioneering studies have shown a crucial correlation between the fat and salt content of food and certain types of cancer and heart disease. Yet, many other diseases are still not associated with diet at all. How could it be that diet, which is responsible for what we are, could not play some sort of role in other degenerative illnesses. And based on the large body of knowledge we do have about the effects of fat, excess salt, sugar, and chemicals, why hasn't there been an informed national program to educate the American public about wiser dietary and hence, health habits?

The result of this nutritional information gap is the willingness of people to try "quack cures." In an attempt to gain some sort of relief from the agonies of different diseases, many are willing to endure what in normal circumstances they would surely laugh at. Yet, this is easy to understand if one has ever faced the prospect of daily pain and suffering without the hope of relief.

Quack cures usually promise instant, miraculous results. They are short-term treatments that do not attempt to reestablish whole-body health. They reflect no knowledge of cause, and most important, they are expensive and usually involve taking exotic ingredients. Overall lifestyle and dietary patterns are not considered, thus precluding the expectation of permanent recovery. The power of our daily food cannot be over-looked in securing our general health and the health of the reproductive system.

Balancing Our Diet

Earlier in this book a chart was given categorizing food according to yin and yang. This information is provided as a guide to understanding the effects various foods exert on our body. The term "effects" refers to the total energetic influence of a food—whether it will have an overall more yang, contracting influence, or a more yin, expanding influence. Eating primarily more yang foods will have a contracting effect on the whole body—physical, emotional, mental, and spiritual. Eating primarily more yin food will have the opposite or expanding effect. Human beings (and all things) need both of these energies. Neither is good or bad. The balance between these two forces, in respect to individual, environmental, and social conditions, is called health. This well-being is a condition in which all body functions, on all levels, operate naturally and appropriately, allowing us to flexibly adjust to any circumstance.

What then does not constitute dietary balance? First, a diet that is unnecessarily narrow, that lacks a wide range of foods, does not represent a balanced dietary plan. Many individuals tend to consume a very limited range of foods. This may be due to taste preference, out of habit, or in the mistaken belief in certain "wonder" foods, that is, foods that have special abilities to prevent illness, or to enhance particular qualities.

Usually this dominant class of foods is from either the extreme yang or extreme yin category. Depending upon an individual's condition, the effects of these imbalanced foods can show up rather quickly or over a longer period of time. Inevitably, however, they will produce bodily imbalances that will appear as symptoms.

From the perspective of yin and yang, whole cereal grains are the most central or balanced food. Thus, in the macrobiotic approach to diet, the proportion of grains and grain products is higher than food from other categories. This is not to diminish the role of other food groups. To the contrary. As just one example, standard macrobiotic dietary suggestions emphasize the consumption of fresh vegetables, served in a variety of ways, in proportions exceeding the daily intake of many people. A quick reading of any macrobiotic cookbook will show the incredible variety of foods and methods of preparation used regularly.

If we consume extreme foods (either yin or yang) on a daily basis, the body's ability to maintain balance will progressively diminish. This is especially true when more centrally or naturally balanced foods are excluded. If our dietary pattern includes both of these extremes, as many people's do, both extreme yin and extreme yang problems will develop.

Extreme foods generate reactions or symptoms that reveal their effects throughout the body. The apparently limitless number of symptoms appearing in widely different parts of the body can be confusing and unsettling for the individual experiencing them. The tendency is to see them as separate problems rather than divergent reactions of a common underlying problem—in this case dietary extremes.

By way of illustration, a diet centered around extreme yin foods, such as simple sugars, certain types of dairy food including ice cream and milk, alcohol, coffee, spices, tropical fruits and vegetables, may produce any of the following symptoms: diarrhea resulting from weak and expanded intestines, poor digestion, a stomach that is easily upset, coughing as the overburdened lungs attempt to discharge excess yin, chronic fatigue as the kidneys weaken, diminished sexual drive and ability, frequent headaches in the front of the head due to expanded nerve and brain cells in that area. This is by no means a complete list. It is provided simply to show the range of problems that can develop from a single cause—excessive yin factors in one's diet.

Conversely, a diet centered around more yang foods such as meat and poultry, eggs, baked foods, and excess salt, can produce any of the following symptoms: constipation caused by intestines that have become too tight, a huge appetite and/or strong cravings, difficulty in breathing due to tightness in the lungs, and headaches more in the back of the head and neck, and in the central part of the head. Again, this limited list of examples is given merely to illustrate the variety of problems that can develop from the same underlying cause.

Individuals consuming extremes from just one side are usually doing so to balance the opposite extreme that has built up in their physical condition and/or in their personal lives. Eventually, they will be attracted to the opposite extreme if serious problems do not develop first. Most people maintain a wide and short-term balance by eating from both extremes.

While traveling recently, I met with some friends in a breakfast shop. It was about 8:30 a.m. and the place was crowded. In most cases, people ordered eggs with either bacon, ham, or sausage. Without exception, they added salt and pepper, and most also used ketchup on their eggs. Afterward they would have coffee with two or three teaspoons of sugar, and milk. Many also had a donut, which seemed to be a speciality of the shop.

How clearly the principle of yin and yang was operating. Eating one extreme required the balancing factor of the opposite extreme. Eggs, fried meats, and salt were balanced by sugar, spices, coffee, and milk. No one can live outside the principles of nature. However, if we make our balance in an unconscious, haphazard manner, we are bound to swing from one extreme to the other.

Such extremes create a variety of symptoms that are caused by extremes of both yin and yang. For example, we may have headaches that start in the back of the head and then move toward the front. Or we may experience alternating bouts of constipation and diarrhea.

Clearly, our way of eating can lead to a variety of symptoms affecting the whole body. Although they may seem unrelated, they are of a common origin.

How We Become What We Eat

The process of digestion starts with the cooking of food. Through the application of heat, the addition of salt, the use of pressure, and adjustments in the lengths of time, cooking begins the breakdown of foods. We can call this stage *preliminary digestion*, or *predigestion*. Its purpose is to make it easier for our bodies to assimilate what we eat.

In the body, digestion begins in the mouth. Chewing mechanically breaks down food and mixes it with the starch-digesting enzymes in the saliva. In the stomach, protein-digesting enzymes and various acids are secreted to continue the digestive process. The *duodenum*, the connection between the stomach and the small intestine, receives digestive enzymes from the pancreas, and bile from the gall bladder. Pancreatic enzymes work on carbohydrates, proteins, and fat. Bile acts on fat.

The breakdown of food is completed in the small intestine. In this warm, dark, moist environment, primitive life, in the form of micro-organisms, reduce the now-digested food to its smallest particles. It is now ready to be absorbed into the body proper by the intestinal villi. How efficiently digestion proceeds depends on the types of food we eat, how we cook them, and the manner in which we eat them (more about the manner of eating later).

This entire process, from cooking through assimilation, returns food to its original state of evolution, that of a single cell. Then the single cell is further broken down into its constituent parts. Digestion thus represents a reversal in the evolutionary process. The easier foods are to break down, the easier it is for our bodies to absorb them. Once absorbed, the opposite process of reassembling, or foreward evolutional development begins—food evolves into our body, our cells, tissues, organs, bones, and so on.

As human beings, we require food that will help us realize our natural status on the evolutionary scale. By eating whole cereal grains as our primary food, we are taking in the segement of the plant kingdom that nourished our emergence as human beings. Other food categories—beans, vegetables, and so on, are secondary to our consumption of cereal grains. If our diet centers around foods from an earlier period of plant evolution—primarily vegetables, or nuts, or fruits, for instance—we are eating lower on the evolutionary scale, thus depriving our body of factors necessary to the development of human beings.

On the other hand, if we eat primarily food from the animal kingdom, especially those near us on the evolutionary ladder, such as cow, pig, or lamb, we are limiting our evolutionary development. Rather than completing the process of human development, we begin to take on the qualities of these lower creatures.

For example, consuming chicken on a daily basis will naturally create a chicken-like influence in our body, emotions, and mind. Eating the foods that influenced the biological evolution of chickens, we also begin to take on chicken-like qualities. This is a natural process that has long been recognized by humanity. In the *Gospel of Thomas*, Christ echoed this point when he said. "Blessed is the lion which becomes man when consumed by man; and cursed is the man whom the lion consumes, and the lion becomes man."

There are thus two ways in which we begin to take on qualities of creatures lower on the biological scale. We can eat a diet that nourished their evolution, or we can eat the creatures themselves.

Although this concept, only briefly outlined here, may seem strange at first, we show unconscious recognition of it in our daily lives. People are often described as having animal-like traits. Someone chatters like a monkey, or behaves like a bull in a china shop, or is as sly as a fox. Someone is an old cow, a snake in the grass, creamy, or fishy. These descriptions depict the biological, mental, and emotional qualities of the person in question. And these characteristics are a direct reflection of the individual's way of eating.

Vegetable-quality foods also create traits which are often recognized in general discussion. When we call someone fruity, nutty, sweet, peachy, oily, or slimy, we are depicting the individual's physical and mental characteristics. These traits emerge as a direct response to the person's dietary orientation.

Actually, all foods have their effect on our total being. Extreme foods have extreme effects, like the ones listed above, which tend to draw attention to themselves. A balanced diet, in harmony with our evolutionary history, environment, and condition, and consisting of grains, vegetables, beans, soups, and occasional seafood, nuts, fruits, and so on, will create a balanced character.

The effects, physical and mental, of eating certain foods, represent the body's adjustment to them. Sickness is simply the body's natural process of becoming—biologically, emotionally, and mentally—what we have been eating.

Most of us know how difficult it can be to make real changes in our lives. Despite our best intentions, too often our attempts end in frustration. This is because we have been playing with shadows, or symptoms, instead of dealing with fundamental issues. Personal growth, as we have seen, begins with the assessment of daily diet.

Currently, about 42 percent of our diet is composed of fat. This has a huge impact on reproductive functions, as well as on overall health. *Dietary Goals for the United States* recommends that Americans reduce overall fat consumption to 30 percent of energy intake. It further suggests that saturated fat should account for no more than 10 percent of total energy intake. Reductions in the incidence of heart disease, cancer, and obesity were some of the expected results of this reduction.

In comparison to the two other macronutrients, carbohydrates and protein, fat is more yin. Fat floats on top of the liquid contents of the stomach, for instance, and during digestion, it leaves the stomach last. Overall, fat contains more of Earth's more upward energy, while the two other nutrients contain more downward energy.

The broad category of fat can be divided into yin fat and yang fat. Yang fat comes from animal sources like beef (hamburger, steak, roast beef), pork (ham, bacon, sausage), chicken, eggs, and hard salty cheeses. This fat is hard, and it remains solid at room temperature. It is more resistant to heat. Yin fat is found in less salty, softer cheeses, liquid dairy products (milk, cream, butter, yogurt), and various oils (sunflower, corn, peanut, olive, sesame). Rather than solidifying at room temperature, yin fats tend to become or remain liquid. They are less resistant to heat and burn easily—put into a hot pan, the more yin fat will quickly start to smoke.

In the duodenum, bile, secreted from the gall bladder, and pancreatic digestive enzymes, *emulsify*, or break down fat into small particles in preparation for assimilation. The bloodstream has a special transport system, called *lipid proteins*, to carry fat. By attaching to these proteins, fat is carried through the blood from the small intestine to the liver. The liver has a limited capacity to store fat Amounts beyond this are sent to various parts of the body for storage. This is a key point. The accumulation and storage of fat in the body leads to a variety of health problems. And, the fact that our current diet contains a large percentage of fat, indicates that these accumulations are common.

Using dairy food as an example, we can see the high-fat content of commonly eaten foods. Cow's milk, 3.5 percent; Half-and-Half, 10.5 percent; Coffee cream, 18 percent; Whipping cream, 30 percent. The fat content of various cheeses is even higher. Cheddar, 34 percent; Parmesan, 28 percent, Romano, 27 percent; Provolone, 28 percent; Blue, 32 percent; and Cottage Cheese, 4 percent.

To understand the movement or distribution of fat in our body, the following classification has been made according to yin and yang.

Yang Fat	*Yin Fat*
Chicken	Softer, less salty cheese
Eggs	Liquid dairy: milk, cream, butter
Beef	Yogurt
Pork	Various oils including vegetable oils
Other meats	Unsaturated fat in general
Hard salty cheeses	
Saturated fat in general	

Yang fats, carried by the bloodstream, tend to go deeper into the body. They primarily affect the deeper body organs such as the kidneys, liver, and heart, and the lower organs in the body, such as intestines, prostate, bladder, ovaries, Fallopian tubes, and uterus. Yang fats tend to gather on the inside organs and can easily condense and solidify.

The more yin fats tend to move toward the body's periphery and towards the external parts of the organs. They also move more toward the upper part of the body. They can easily overburden the lymph system.

Foods high in fat cannot be properly digested or assimilated. Instead they become excess that is distributed and stored in various parts of the body according to their yin and yang quality. It is easy to see this process taking place in the sexual organs.

The reproductive system is located in the lower torso, a more downward or yang area in general. Some areas, however, are more inner or centrally located, while others are more peripheral. In the male reproductive system, the more yang fats tend to gather and condense in the central areas of the prostate and bladder. Whereas the more yin fats tend to accumulate in peripheral areas such as the testes and the network of tubes connecting the testes to the urinary tract. In each case there can be both yin and yang fat but the proportion is different.

In the female reproductive tract the more yang fats tend to gather and condense on the inside of the uterus, the ovaries, and the Fallopian tubes. The more yin fats tend to accumulate on the periphery of the uterus, ovaries, tubes, and in the vaginal region. Again, both yin and yang fats may be found, but their proportion and exact location will differ.

This accumulation of yin and yang fat can be given names, such as cyst, lump, tumor, or endometriosis. In the male it may be called varicocele, blockage of the tubes or the ducts, or hardening or enlargement of the prostate. These names simply reflect the location and identifying characteristics of the accumulation. They should not be allowed to disguise their basic cause. We are becoming what we eat.

Diet and Reproductive Health

As we have seen, all things contain both yin and yang factors. The human reproductive system is no exception. Both sexes need a good balance of yin and yang foods, concentrating on the central area of grains, beans, vegetables, and so on, and avoiding the extremes of both categories. The quality of these foods is of course crucial. For our reproductive system to work as it should, we need foods that have life and vitality. To increase our fertility, we need foods that are fertile.

Whole cereal grains are capable of producing new plants if put into the ground. Beans and seeds can do the same. Fresh vegetables are full of life. The life-giving property of the foods we eat increases our own life-giving ability. On the other hand, we diminish our vitality and our fertility when we eat denatured, processed, sterilized, and chemically preserved foods.

Within the overall balance of yin and yang foods, males and females respectively need a balance appropriate to their own unique natures. The basic complementary/antagonistic relationship between male and female must be considered when establishing sound dietary patterns.

Males, as explained previously, are created and nurtured more by Heaven's centripetal force. Masculine characteristics, physical and mental, are a reflection of this influence. More specifically, the structure and function of the male reproductive system, as we have seen, is nourished by this downward, contracting tendency. Foods carrying this same energy pattern reinforce this male-type orientation.

Thus, within the overall category of a centrally balanced diet, men will use slightly more of the foods that provide this centripetal energy. How much depends on many factors, including climate, season, locale, age, condition, occupation, and so on. Although this may seem complicated, with the use of the Unifying Principles of yin and yang, it becomes clear that such adjustments are nothing more than common sense.

Examples of such food items include buckwheat, root vegetables, seafood, and slightly stronger condiments. A food's energy is also affected by how it is prepared. By adjusting the use of salt and salt products, pressure, cooking times, and the strength of the flame, dishes can be more strongly energized. These and other factors are explained in detail in the companion to this book, *Infertility and Reproductive Disorders*, in the *Macrobiotic Food and Cooking Series*.

It is important to remember that men should not ignore the good-quality yin foods. Rather, within an overall balanced diet containing both yin and yang items, men can select occasional side dishes that are compatible to their basic energetic orientation.

Females are created and nurtured more by Earth's centrifugal force. Feminine characteristics, including the structure and function of the female reproductive system, reflect this upward-moving, expanding energy. Consequently, within an overall balanced way of eating, females can use slightly more of the foods that provide centrifugal energy. Again, to what degree such foods are emphasized depends on a variety of environmental and personal variables.

Example of foods that provide this type of energy include lightly cooked green leafy vegetables, occasional raw salads and fruit, fermented foods, and grain sweeteners. Preparation styles using less time, a lower flame, less pressure, fermentation, and less salt and salt products, enhance this type of energy.

This is not to say that females should avoid the more yang type foods. It implies instead that within the overall dietary pattern, the balance leans toward the use of good-quality yin foods.

Diet and Male Reproductive Health ━━━━━━━━

The influence of centripetal or yang energy in the mature male body creates a strong, healthy sexual drive, the ability to have and sustain an erection, the ability to ejaculate, the production of healthy sperm cells in the testes, and the production of male hormones. When energy flows smoothly through the body, male desire and ability in sexual intercourse is healthy and strong.

Characteristic effects of Heaven's force in the male body include the gathering or concentrating in the reproductive system of such forces as blood and other body fluids, cells, and the production of heat. When an excessive amount of the opposite energy is taken in, in the form of items like sugar, chocolate, fruits and fruit juices—especially those of tropical origin—alcohol, drugs, and light dairy food—milk, sweetened yogurt, cream, butter—this gathering of male sexual energy is dispersed.

There is an interesting paradox here. Initially, extreme yin food seems to stimulate sexual desire. This happens as the concentrated energy is released by the expansive effects of such items. Over time, however, this store of concentrated energy will be depleted, and sexual ability will decrease. If continued, this dietary practice can lead to difficulties in attaining an erection, and in extreme cases, impotence. In the short-term, the production of healthy sperm will decrease. Their shape may change to double-tailed, or split mitochondria, and the number of immature sperm cells may increase. Their vitality and motility can be weakened.

The production of the pituitary hormones FSH and LH, which are influenced by Heaven's downward force, may be lowered. In extreme cases this could be diminished to the point that the hormonal cycle cannot operate properly and the production of testosterone will not be adequate to sustain basic male characteristics. The prostate and bladder will also be affected. The prostate can become enlarged resulting in diminished efficiency of its secretions. The bladder can become swollen, with potential problems in urination.

The intricate network of tubes through which sperm are created and must travel can become loose and accumulate fat. The blood quality nourishing the reproductive system tends to become acidic, making the reproductive system vulnerable to various infections. The resultant scarring that may occur can cause serious problems with fertility.

Related mental and emotional problems can accompany these biological problems. There can be nervousness, anxiety, avoidance of sexual situations, self-doubt, and depression. Mood swings can lead to irritability and unstable behavior patterns.

In the opposite case, a diet composed of extreme yang foods, such as eggs, meats, salty foods, poultry, shellfish, and hard salty cheeses, will excessively stimulate the downward flow of Heaven's force in the male body. Despite the fact that these foods stimulate male sexual energy, they are extreme yang, and when taken on a regular basis, they contract and constrict the male reproductive system to an excessive degree. Because these foods all have a high fat content, accumulations and blockages can develop.

Extreme yang foods impede the production of healthy sperm. Their shape and motility will be affected. The intricate network of tubes through which sperm travel can easily accumulate fat and become blocked. When this occurs there is a buildup of heat in the scrotal area that can kill sperm.

With the storage of so much salt and fat not only in the reproductive system, but throughout the body, the hormonal cycle can be impaired. Excess fat can block the proper secretion of the pituitary gland, thus inhibiting proper secretion of FSH, LH, and also testosterone.

The prostate gland can accumulate fat and become enlarged and hardened, damaging fertility. The bladder can also have a fat buildup which adversely affects urination.

The mental and emotional counterpart of these biological disorders can be a feeling of tension, inability to express oneself, repression and occasional outbursts in order to release this built-up frustration and anger.

In most cases there is a combination of both extremes eaten, resulting in a combination of symptoms throughout the body, including the reproductive tract. Depending on which way the diet tilts, either more yin or yang, will determine the particular set of symptoms in a given individual.

The surest, quickest way to weaken the reproductive system is to follow such a dietary pattern. The effect of long-time eating of both extremes can be overcome by understanding that we are responsible for our own health and well-being and that we have the power to control it by our way of eating and way of life.

Diet and Female Reproductive Health ────────

Since females are nourished more by foods and cooking styles with Earth's upward energy, the opposite or downward-moving energy, if taken in extremes, is most damaging to female reproductive health. Examples of extreme yang foods include: eggs, meats, salty foods, harder saltier cheeses, poultry (including chicken and turkey), shellfish, and long-time baked foods. If such items are consumed daily over an extended period of time, the female reproductive tract will become too tight and constricted. And because of the high fat content in these foods there will be excess, accumulation, and blockage.

Fat accumulations in the ovaries, Fallopian tubes, and uterus, can lead to problems with egg production and ovulation. The Fallopian tubes can narrow with the accumulation of fat and twists or kinks can arise, blocking the passage of the egg to the uterus and the movement of sperm toward the egg. Inside the uterus, fat accumulation can lead to lumps and tumors, either benign or cancerous. The menstrual cycle can be altered, possibly shortened, and menstruation itself can be painful. In the extreme, menstruation can stop altogether.

Along with these internal changes, the possibility for infection increases. Although generally localized, infections can spread throughout the system. As a result, scarring can occur due to the inability to heal properly.

When this way of extreme eating is combined with the use of oral contraceptives, the reproductive system and the hormonal system are both thrown out of balance. Birth control pills, which are synthetic hormones, change the alternating hormonal secretions between the pituitary and the sexual organs. This natural balance, responding to the body's needs at any given time, is essential not only for reproductive health, but the well-being of the whole body.

The insertion of a foreign object into the body for contraceptive purposes can lead to the gathering of fat around it. The body's natural reaction is to neutralize or eliminate it. The use of various contraceptive devices and sprays change the delicate chemical balance of the fluids of the reproductive system. This can cause numerous reproductive problems and weaken fertility.

The endocrine system can be blocked because of fat, and its secretions diminished or, in the extreme, totally blocked. The production of FSH and LH, and estrogen and progesterone can be altered and their delicate balance upset.

Mental and emotional symptoms of an extremely yang dietary pattern can be varied. Examples include irritability and anger, tension from the improper functioning of the menstrual cycle, especially the proper discharge and repair of the endometrial lining.

A diet of extreme yin foods will also cause female reproductive problems. Although the energy of these foods carries more of Earth's force, they are extreme and thus have extremely yin effects on the body. They can loosen the reproductive system, weaken blood quality, and easily turn to fat in the body.

The production of one strong egg by the ovary will be affected, often weakening the egg or causing the secretion of more than one egg. If this is continued, egg production could stop altogether. Various cysts and accumulations can form on the outside of the ovary. The Fallopian tubes can be covered with fat that can block vital blood flow and impede the passage of an egg and sperm. The outside of the uterus can be covered with fat which can easily spread to other areas throughout the reproductive system.

Overall, the body will become colder and weaker from this extreme type of eating, and the result could be diminished or total lack of interest in sex. Because the quality of the blood nourishing the reproductive area tends to become acidic, the chance for infections of various kinds is greatly increased. These can easily spread throughout the reproductive tract and scarring can result.

The hormonal balance will be impaired with the production of FSH and LH, greatly weakened, and in the extreme, totally stopped. As a result, the menstrual cycle can be delayed, leading to the incomplete discharge of the endometrial tissue during menstruation can be reduced.

Mentally, this can lead to anxiety, tension and nervousness. Depression can alternate with hyperactivity as the blood-sugar level radically jumps from highs to lows.

In the case where both extremes are eaten, there can be a combination of symptoms. The predominance of a given symptom will depend on which way the diet tilts, toward more yang or more yin.

Physical, mental, and emotional symptoms have their origin in our daily eating. If a diet of extremes is continued for an extended period of time, these symptoms can require continued medication and the possibility of surgery to remove troubled areas. Although these methods may be used as symptomatic treatments, if the cause is not changed, new or similar problems will develop. Without understanding and distinguishing between cause—lifestyle and diet—and effects—sickness, and symptoms—the health of the reproductive system cannot truly be reestablished.

5.   The Macrobiotic Approach━━━

By definition, the macrobiotic approach to well-being begins from
a large view. From the Greek *makro* (large) and *bios* (life), and
meaning "large or long life," macrobiotics can be literally defined as
"living according to a large view of life." By understanding individual
phenomenon in relation to the whole, by seeing the dynamics of cause
and effect at work in any particular example, and by being aware of
long-term as well as short-term implications, macrobiotics is a practical and effective tool for personal and social growth.

Within the macrobiotic approach, any steps to relieve infertility or
reproductive disorders begin with reestablishing total health. In
many cases, simply adopting standard macrobiotic dietary patterns
will produce profound improvements in overall well-being. This in
itself reveals the origin of ill health as extreme dietary practice. However, the importance of other lifestyle factors should not be over-
looked. More will be said about this aspect later on.

It is important to remember that the Standard Macrobiotic Diet is
not a diet in the usual sense of the word. Instead, it is a set of general
guidelines within which there is an incredible amount of variety and
flexibility for personal choice. Individuals are free to make adjustments as their conditions and circumstances dictate. Also, the
"standard diet" varies according to environmental conditions,
including climate and season. We are not describing a one-month
crash plan, but a life-long change in dietary and lifestyle habits that
will help us to maintain well-being as long as we live. Let us now
examine in detail the incredible variety of foods that are included in a
macrobiotic way of eating.

The Standard Macrobiotic Way of Eating━━━

The standard macrobiotic way of eating has been practiced throughout
history by all major cultures. In modern times it has often been
misunderstood due to a lack of factual dietary information and basic
understanding of the traditional dietary practices of cultures based
on the order of nature.

Macrobiotic eating is very broad. It has been practiced by hundreds
of thousands of people, especially in the last 15 years—people wishing
to attain better health and create well-being within their families and
society.

Fig. 15

This chart shows macrobiotic dietary recommendations. The proportions provide a general guideline for daily eating.

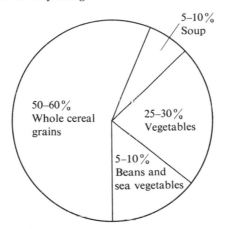

Plus condiments and beverages
Occasional use: Fish and seafoods
Seasonal fruits
Nuts, seeds, and other natural snacks

The macrobiotic way of eating is similar in orientation to the dietary guidelines issued by the following public health agencies:

- The United States Congress, Senate Select Committee on Nutrition and Human Needs publication, *Dietary Goals for the United States* (1976).
- The U. S. Surgeon General's report, *Healthy People: Health Promotion and Disease Prevention* (1979).
- Dietary guidelines issued by the American Heart Association, The American Diabetes Association, The American Society for Clinical Nutrition, and the U. S. Department of Agriculture.
- A 1981 report by a panel of the American Association for the Advancement of Science.
- The dietary guidelines for cancer prevention issued by the National Academy of Sciences in the 1982 report, *Diet, Nutrition, and Cancer.*
- Dietary guidelines issued by the American Cancer Society (1984).

The standard macrobiotic way of eating is not intended for any particular person nor for a particular disease. It is designed for the purpose of maintaining physical and psychological health and the well-being of society in general. It further serves in many instances to prevent degenerative diseases and promote possible recovery from disorders.

The guidelines presented below are appropriate for people living in a temperate four-season climate. Modifications are required for people in a tropical and sub-tropical climate, as well as those in polar and semi-polar regions.

The macrobiotic way of eating is derived from the principles presented previously. For example, it:

- Considers human needs within the order of biological life.
- Respects centuries' old dietary customs from cultures throughout the world.
- Can be readily adapted to climatic, seasonal, and environmental differences.
- Considers social and economic requirements and can be practiced widely throughout the world at a reasonable cost.
- Satisfies the nutritional balance and basic requirements for human needs.

We will now examine each of the food categories in the standard macrobiotic way of eating in detail.

Whole Grains

Within the standard macrobiotic way of eating and especially in a temperate climate, whole grains are an essential part of the daily diet. They comprise 40 to 60 percent (average 50 percent) of daily food intake.

Kinds of Whole Grains and Grain Products
Brown Rice
    Brown rice—short, medium, and long grain
    Genuine brown rice cream
    Puffed brown rice
    Brown rice flour products
    Brown rice flakes
Sweet Brown Rice
    Sweet brown rice grain
    Mochi (pounded sweet brown rice)
    Sweet brown rice flour products
Wild Rice
    Wild rice grain

Whole Wheat
  Whole wheat berries
  Whole wheat bread
  Whole wheat chapatis
  Whole wheat noodles and pasta
  Whole wheat flakes
  Whole wheat flour products, such as crackers, matzos, muffins,
    and others
  Couscous
  Bulgur
  Fu (baked puffed wheat gluten)
  Seitan (wheat gluten)
Barley
  Barley grain
  Pearl barley
  Pearled barley
  Puffed barley
  Barley flour products
Rye
  Rye grain
  Rye bread
  Rye flakes
  Rye flour products
Millet
  Millet grain
  Millet flour products
  Puffed millet
Oats
  Whole oats
  Steel-cut oats
  Rolled oats
  Oatmeal
  Oat flakes
  Oat flour products and puffed oats
Corn
  Corn on the cob
  Corn grits
  Corn meal
  Arepas
  Corn flour products such as corn bread, muffins, etc.
  Puffed corn
  Popped corn
Buckwheat

Buckwheat groats
Buckwheat noodles and pasta
Buckwheat flour products such as pancakes, etc.
Other Traditional Grains
Such as triticale, etc.

Soup

The macrobiotic way of eating recommends, under normal circumstances, an average consumption of two cups or bowls of soup each day.

Kinds of Soup
Light broth for noodles or pasta
Vegetable soup
Vegetable and sea vegetable (usually *wakame* or *kombu*) soup
Bean and vegetable soup
Grain and vegetable soup
Fish and vegetable soup
Fish, vegetable, and sea vegetable soup
Noodle vegetable soup
Mochi and vegetable soup
Bread and vegetable soup
Dumpling and vegetable soup
Stew with grains, vegetables, beans, sea vegetables and/or fish and seafood
Other traditionally used soups
Seasonings for Soup
Miso (fermented soybean and grain paste)
Tamari soy sauce (fermented soybean and grain soy sauce)
Sea salt
Sesame or corn oil (occasionally)
Other traditionally used condiments

Vegetables

A wide selection of vegetable dishes prepared in a variety of cooking styles may comprise approximately 30 percent of daily food intake.

Kinds of Vegetables	Burdock root	Celery
Acorn squash	Buttercup squash	Celery root
Bok choy	Butternut squash	Carrots
Broccoli	Cabbage	Carrot tops

Cauliflower	*Jinenjo*	Scallions
Chinese cabbage	Jerusalem artichoke	*Shiitake* mushrooms
Chives	Kale	Snap beans
Collard greens	Kohlrabi	Summer squash
Coltsfoot	Leeks	Turnip greens
Cucumber	Lotus root	Watercress
Daikon	Lamb's-quarters	Wax beans
Daikon Greens	Mushrooms	Winter melon
Dandelion leaves	Mustard greens	Wild grasses that
Dandelion roots	Onion	have been used
Endive	Parsley	widely for centuries
Escarole	Parsnip	Other vegetables that
Green beans	Pumpkin	have been tradi-
Green peas	Patty pan squash	tionally used and
Hokkaido pumpkin	Radish	commonly consumed
Hubbard squash	Red cabbage	
Iceberg lettuce	Romaine lettuce	

Beans

The standard macrobiotic way of eating recommends regular consumption of beans and bean products. Beans may comprise 5 to 10 percent of daily food intake.

Kinds of Beans

Azuki beans	Navy beans
Black-eyed peas	Pinto beans
Black turtle beans	Soybeans
Black soybeans	Split peas
Chick-peas (garbanzo beans)	Whole dried peas
Great northern beans	Bean sprouts
Kidney beans	Other beans which have
Lentils	been traditionally used
Lima beans	
Mung beans	

Kinds of Bean Products
Dried *tofu* (soybean curd that has been dried)
Fresh tofu
Okara (residue in making tofu)
Natto (fermented soybeans)
Tempeh (fermented soybeans)

Sea Vegetables

The standard macrobiotic way of eating recommends sea vegetables be consumed daily or frequently as side dishes or in the preparation of other foods. Sea vegetables may comprise a small percentage of daily intake.

Kinds of Sea Vegetables
Arame	*Nekabu*
Agar-agar	*Nori*
Dulse	Wakame
Hijiki	Other sea vegetables that
Irish moss (sea moss)	have traditionally been used
Kombu	
Mekabu	

Fish and Seafood

The standard macrobiotic way of eating recommends fish and seafood as an occasional supplement to the above categories of food—grains, soups, vegetables, beans, and beverages. The amount of fish or seafood can vary according to personal needs and can range from once in a while to several times a week. The average, however, is twice or three times a week—with the amount not exceeding 20 percent of the total volume of food consumed that day. The kinds of fish and seafood recommended are those with less saturated fat and those which are most easily digested.

Kinds of Fish and Seafood
Carp	Herring
Cod	Scrod
Dried fish	Smelt
Small dried fish (*iriko*)	Snapper
Flounder	Sole
Haddock	Trout
Halibut	White-meat fish

Seafood Used Occasionally
Cherrystone clams	Octopus
Littleneck clams	Oysters
Clams	Lobster
Crab	Shrimp

Infrequently Used Fish, not preferred for regular use
Bluefish	Salmon

Sardines	Other blue-skinned or red-meat
Swordfish	fish
Tuna	

Fruit

The standard macrobiotic way of eating includes occasional consumption of fruit, depending upon climate, season, personal need, and circumstances. All traditionally used and commonly consumed fruits growing in a temperate climate are included. The regular use of tropical fruits in a temperate climate is not recommended.

Kinds of Fruit

Apples	Plums
Apricots	Raisins
Blackberries	Raspberries
Cantaloupe	Strawberries
Grapes	Tangerines
Grapefruit	Watermelon
Honeydew melon	Wild berries
Lemons	Other fruit traditionally grown
Mulberries	in a temperate climate
Oranges	
Persimmon	
Peaches	

Variety of Serving Styles for Fruit
Fresh and raw
Fresh, raw, and soaked in lightly salted water
Grated
Boiled
Baked
Steamed
Juice as a beverage or flavoring
Preserves
Spread on bread or other baked-flour products
As an ingredient in stuffing
As a dessert
As an ingredient and flavoring in *kuzu* or agar-agar gelatin
Baked in bread
Dried fruit as a snack, garnish, or dessert
Pickled fruit
Deep-fried fruit (in a batter)
Served as a garnish

96

Fermented beverages
Other traditionally used and commonly consumed serving styles

Pickles

The standard macrobiotic way of eating recommends frequent use of
pickles as a supplement to various main dishes for the purpose of
stimulating appetite and encouraging digestion. Some pickles are
available in natural food stores, while many can be prepared at home.
Some are ready in a few hours, others require more time—from a few
days to a few seasons.

Kinds of Food Often Used in Making Pickles

Anchovies	Lotus root
Apricots	Mustard greens
Burdock root	Olives
Broccoli	Onions
Cabbage	Pumpkin
Carrots	Radishes, red and white
Cauliflower	Red cabbage
Caviar	Scallions
Chinese cabbage	Squash
Cucumbers	Turnips
Daikon	Salmon
Herring	Sardines
Leeks	Other foods traditionally used for making pickles

Methods Used in Pickling
  Brine pickles
  Bran pickles
  Miso pickles
  Pressed pickles
  Salt and water pickles
  Salt pickles
  Sauerkraut
  Takuan pickles
  Tamari soy sauce pickles
  Umeboshi pickles
  Other traditionally used and commonly practiced pickling methods

Nuts

The standard macrobiotic way of eating can include occasional consumption of various kinds of nuts in the form of snacks, garnishes, or as an ingredient in desserts.

Kinds of Nuts
  Almonds
  Chestnuts
  Filberts
  Peanuts

  Pecans
  Pinenuts
  Small Spanish nuts
  Walnuts

Less Frequently Used Nuts
  Brazil nuts
  Cashews
  Macadamia nuts

  Other traditionally used nuts

Seeds

The standard macrobiotic way of eating includes occasional consumption of seeds prepared in a variety of ways.

Kinds of Seeds
  Alfalfa seeds
  Black sesame seeds
  Plum seeds
  Poppy seeds
  Pumpkin seeds
  Squash seeds

  Sunflower seeds
  Umeboshi plum seeds
  White sesame seeds
  Other traditionally used and
      commonly consumed seeds

Serving Styles for Seeds
  As Condiments:
    Dried and ground
    Roasted and ground
    Roasted and ground with sea salt
    With umeboshi powder and sea salt
    With miso
  As Snacks:
    Dried and served alone
    Roasted and served alone
    Baked with flour products such as cookies, crackers, breads,
      cakes, and other baked-flour products
    As an ingredient in candies
    Other traditionally used and commonly consumed snacks

As Garnishes—sprinkled on various dishes such as:

grains	fish and seafood
soups	fruit
vegetable dishes	desserts
beans	

Seasonings Commonly Used with Seeds
Sea salt
Tamari soy sauce
Miso
Barley malt
Rice malt
Other traditionally used and commonly consumed seasonings

Snacks

The standard macrobiotic way of eating includes daily or occasional use of a variety of natural snacks consumed in moderate amounts.

Kinds of Snacks
Grain-based Snacks:
Cookies, crackers, wafers, pancakes, muffins, bread, puffed brown rice, barley, oats, millet, corn, popcorn
Mochi
Noodles and pasta
Rice balls
Rice cakes
Homemade *sushi*
Roasted grains
Other traditionally used and commonly consumed natural snacks
Bean-based Snacks:
Roasted beans
Boiled beans
Nut-based Snacks:
Nuts roasted and seasoned with sea salt
Nuts roasted and seasoned with tamari soy sauce
Nuts roasted and seasoned with barley malt
Nuts roasted and seasoned with rice malt
Nuts used in cookies, crackers, and as an ingredient in other baked-flour products

Condiments

The standard macrobiotic way of eating includes a wide variety of condiments for daily, regular, or occasional use. They are sprinkled on or added in small amounts to food to adjust taste and nutritional value of food and to help stimulate appetite. Condiments are commonly used for grains, soups, vegetables dishes, bean dishes, and sometimes with desserts.

Kinds of Condiments
   Gomashio (roasted sesame seeds and sea salt)
   Sea vegetable powder
   Sea vegetable powder with roasted sesame seeds
   Tekka (condiment made from soybean miso, sesame oil, burdock, lotus root, carrots, and ginger root)
   Umeboshi plum
   Umeboshi plum and raw scallions or onions
   Shio kombu (kombu cooked with tamari soy sauce and water)
   Chopped *shiso* leaves (pickled beefsteak-plant leaves)
   Roasted shiso leaves
   Green nori
   Yellow mustard (used mainly for fish and seafood)
   Green mustard (used mainly for fish and seafood)
   Cooked miso with scallions or onions
   Cooked nori condiment
   Roasted sesame seeds
   Other traditionally used and commonly consumed condiments

Seasonings

The standard macrobiotic way of eating includes regular and occasional use of a variety of seasonings in cooking and before serving. The seasonings are all vegetable-quality and are naturally processed. These seasonings have been used traditionally throughout the world. The use of seasonings can be moderate yet adequate for personal needs.

Kinds of Seasonings
   Unrefined sea salt
   Soy sauce
   Tamari soy sauce
   Miso

Types of Miso
   Rice miso
   Barley miso
   Soybean miso
   Sesame miso
   Other traditionally used and commonly consumed misos
Note: Dark miso has been fermented for a longer period of time.
          Light miso has been fermented for a shorter period of time.

Rice vinegar	Lemon juice
Brown rice vinegar	Tangerine juice
Umeboshi vinegar	Orange juice
Sauerkraut brine	Red pepper
Barley malt	Green mustard paste
Rice malt	Yellow mustard paste
Grated ginger root	Sesame oil
Grated daikon	Corn oil
Grated radish	Safflower oil
Horseradish	Mustard seed oil
Umeboshi paste	Olive oil
Umeboshi plum	

Mirin (sweet cooking wine)
Amazaké (fermented sweet brown rice beverage)
Freshly-ground black pepper
Saké lees (residue in making saké)
Saké (fermented rice wine)
Other natural seasonings which have been traditionally used

Garnishes

The standard macrobiotic way of eating emphasizes balance of
qualities, tastes, nutritional factors, and energetic harmony. For that
purpose, garnishes are used in small amounts to balance some dishes,
especially for the purpose of creating easier digestion.

Kinds of Garnishes
   Grated daikon—used mainly as a garnish for the following:
      Fish and seafood
      Mochi
      Buckwheat noodles and pasta
      Natto
      Tempeh
   Grated radish—used mainly as a garnish for the following:
      same as above

Grated Horseradish—used mainly as a garnish for the following:
   same as above
Chopped scallions—used mainly as a garnish for the following:
   Noodle and pasta dishes
   Fish and seafood
   Natto
   Tempeh
The following:
   Grated ginger   Freshly ground pepper
   Green mustard paste   Lemon pieces
may be used mainly as a garnish for:
   Soup
   Noodle and pasta dishes
   Fish and seafood
The following:
   Red pepper
   Freshly ground pepper
   Green mustard paste
may be used mainly as a garnish for:
   Soup
   Noodle and pasta dishes
   Fish and seafood
   Natto
   Tempeh

Desserts

The standard macrobiotic way of eating includes frequent use of
a variety of desserts usually served at the end of the main meal.

Kinds of Desserts
   Azuki beans sweetened with barley malt or rice malt
   Azuki beans cooked with chestnuts
   Azuki beans cooked with squash
   Kuzu sweetened with barley malt, rice malt, fresh fruit, or dried
      fruit
   Agar-agar cooked with barley malt, rice malt, fresh fruit, or
      dried fruit
   Cooked fruit
   Dried fruit
   Fruit pies including apple, peach, strawberry, berry, and other
      temperate climate fruits
   Fruit crunch including apple, peach, strawberry, berry, and other

temperate climate fruits

Grain desserts sweetened with dried fruits, barley malt, rice malt, amasaké, fresh fruit

Examples of grain desserts: Couscous cake, Indian pudding, rice pudding, and other similar naturally sweetened desserts

Baked-flour desserts such as cookies, cakes, pies, muffins, breads, and others prepared with natural sweeteners including fruits and grain sweeteners

Beverages

The standard macrobiotic way of eating includes a variety of beverages for daily, regular, or occasional consumption. The amount of beverage intake varies according to individual needs and climate change. Beverages comfortably satisfy the desire for liquid in terms of kind, volume, and frequency of intake.

Kinds of Beverages
Bancha twig tea
Bancha stem tea
Roasted rice with bancha twig tea
Roasted barley with bancha twig tea
Kombu tea
Spring water
100-percent cereal grain coffee
Amazaké
Dandelion tea
Lotus root tea
Soybean milk
Burdock root tea
Mu tea
Other traditionally used non-stimulating, non-aromatic natural herb teas (made from seeds, leaves, stems, bark, or roots)
Alcoholic beverages:
Saké—more naturally fermented quality
Beer of various kinds—more naturally fermented quality
Wines of various kinds—more naturally fermented quality
Other grain and fruit-based, weak alcoholic beverages that have been fermented naturally
Fruit juice:
Apple juice
Grape juice

Apricot juice
Cider
Vegetable juice:
Carrot juice
Celery juice
Juice from leafy green vegetables
Beet juice
Barley green juice
Other juices made from vegetables that have been traditionally
grown in temperate climates

Additional Foods

In some instances, such as occasional requirement for nutritional
balance or for special social events, the standard macrobiotic way of
eating can be temporarily modified to include some other foods such
as salmon, tuna, other red-meat, blue-skinned, and fatty fish, organic
fertilized fowl's eggs, caviar, and other fish eggs, white-meat poultry,
skim cow's milk or goat's milk, traditionally fermented cheese and
yogurt, unrefined honey, maple syrup, and beet sugar.

These modifications are made according to individual requirements
and necessity; though within the usual standard macrobiotic way of
eating, these foods are not regularly or commonly required to maintain health and well-being.

The Manner of Eating ━━━━━━━━━━━━━━━━━━━━━━

To establish well-being, macrobiotic eating includes the following
daily practices:

- Eat regularly. Two to three meals a day can be consumed. In the
  case of vigorous physical labor, the frequency of meals can be
  increased to four times a day.
- Include grain or grain products at every meal. Grain and grain
  products can represent 50 percent, more or less, of the daily intake
  of food.
- Variety in the selection and preparation of food, proper combinations, and the correct way of cooking food are essential.
- Cooking is to be done with a peaceful mind, with love, and with
  care.
- Snacks are to be taken only in moderate amounts. They should
  not replace a regular meal.

- Beverages can be consumed comfortably as one desires.
- Refrain from eating before bedtime, preferably 3 hours, except in unusual circumstances.
- Chew very well. Chew each mouthful until it is liquid.
- The volume of food can vary depending upon each individual's needs.
- Eat with the spirit of gratitude and appreciation for people, society, nature, and the universe.

In order to gain a broader perspective of the macrobiotic approach to diet, four crucial areas can be examined.

Historical Reaosns

Historically we find that humanity has consumed cereal grains as its major food. Whole cereals are the most abundant of crops; about one-half the cultivated land in the world is used for growing grains. Whole cereal grains are easily stored and are thus capable of sustaining health and vitality in times of scarcity. For these reasons, grains naturally became the center of humanity's diet. Due to different environmental conditions, various geographical areas developed their own major grain. In the Americas, corn was grown and consumed daily. In the Far East, rice is the major grain. In Europe, wheat, oats, and millet were eaten. In Russia, a colder-climate country, buckwheat was the primary grain. India grew rice and barley.

If we study a particular region of the globe we find that traditionally the peoples of that area had a principal grain food and a cuisine, using local beans and seasonal vegetables, built around it. The eating of animal food was limited to special holidays during the year and during times of extreme cold and scarcity.

The importance of grain cannot be overemphasized. The Encyclopedia Britannica states, "Each of the world's great civilizations has depended upon cereals as a major source of food, being by far man's most important source of carbohydrate. When ancient man learned to grown cereals, he was able to produce more than enough food for his own immediate needs, thus making possible settled communities and the development of the arts and sciences that distinguish civilized man from the savage." In this sense, cereal grains reflect the development of civilization and humanity.

Economic Reasons ━━━━━━━━━━━━━━━━━━━━━━━━━━━

With such an abundance of whole cereal grains it would seem that
food should be plentiful—enough for everyone on the planet—and
the cost should be relatively low. Obviously, this is not the case.
Food costs are high and continue to rise, while malnourishment, even
in wealthy nations, seems to be increasing. Why is this so?

Instead of eating whole grains as a principal food, most modern
societies feed grain to animals, and then eat parts of those animals.
In dollar-and-cents terms, this is a poor business practice. Although
estimates vary, it takes between ten and twenty pounds of grain to
produce one pound of consumable animal protein.

The additional costs of this eating strategy must also be considered.
Examples include the cost of: health-care and inspection of the
animals, transporting, slaughtering, processing, refrigeration, and
packaging.

Since scientific and medical findings have shown a link between
animal-food consumption and various diseases, such as heart disease
and certain types of cancer, we could also factor in the medical costs
that result from such an unbalanced diet.

The same type of reasoning holds true for many other so-called
foods that we commonly eat. Instead of consuming fresh vegetables
and fruits, we process and refine them, adding to their cost, reducing
their nutritional value, and adding harmful preservatives to maintain
shelf-life. Even from a view limited to economic considerations, this
makes no sense. In the economic long- and short-run, macrobiotics
as applied to food production and dietary practices is really our most
intelligent strategy.

Nutritional Factors ━━━━━━━━━━━━━━━━━━━━━━━━━

Although we have touched on nutritional factors before, their importance deserves more attention. Currently our diet tends to be high in
fat, from excessive consumption of animal products and dairy foods,
high in chemical additives, salt, cholesterol, refined foods, and simple
sugars. Little thought is given to an overall dietary plan for lifetime
health.

The body's most important nutritional requirement is carbohydrate.
Our brain and nervous system need a constant supply of carbohydrate—it is the only type of fuel they use. Whole grains supply
carbohydrate in its complex form; a form that evenly sustains our
energy needs over an extended period of time. Simple sugars, on the

other hand, tend to increase our sugar level dramatically, and then to drop it just as fast, leaving us physically and emotionally depleted.

When we eat whole cereal grains, we receive a generous supply of fiber, that keeps our intestines functioning efficiently. Grains also contain protein, roughly 7 to 12 percent, and in their outer hull, carry vitamins and minerals. Of course we eat a large variety of other foods in addition to grains. Because they are in their whole and natural state, their nutritional content is varied and high.

Many current "diets" emphasize one dietary aspect at the expense of others. Examples include those diets that concentrate on protein, or a particular mineral, vitamin, or enzyme. These factors are of course important, but within a total nutritional picture, rather than in concentrated or isolated amounts. Our basic sense tells us that we want total or complete health, and to accomplish this we should consider all of our body's nutritional needs. This is why macrobiotics is a most balanced and reasonable way of eating for health and happiness.

Biological Reasons

The plant kingdom is the primary means by which the animal kingdom adapts, evolves, and sustains itself. Any change that took place in the plant kingdom during evolution was mirrored in the animal kingdom. This ongoing process has culminated in the most modern evolutionary product of the plant world—the cereal grain plant—and in the most modern evolutionary product of the animal world—human beings. Humanity has achieved its status because of grains, and the continued consumption of grains sustains and enhances it.

We are a blueprint of biological evolution, a living representation of all the stages that unfolded over the several billion years of evolution. There is a dietary strategy that allows us to account for and nourish all past biological stages in our eating. Within macrobiotic guidelines there are: various fermented foods representing the diverse bacteria from which all higher forms of life originated; soup which is a replica of the ancient ocean from which we evolved; sea vegetables representing the period when the earth was covered by water; land vegetables, both large leafy vegetables showing the time when earth was subject to a warmer climate, and smaller, more compact vegetables representing a time when the earth's climate was cooling; beans, seeds, and nuts, representing the evolutionary period prior to cereal grains; and finally, whole cereal grains, our opposite and complementary partner in the evolutionary process. Grains are our evolutionary parent and therefore make up a large portion of our diet.

This way of eating nourishes, in proper proportion, the past biological stages that we carry in our human body. We select primarily from the plant kingdom because it is the source of animal life and evolution. By eating this way we are able to fully realize our normal human status of health and happiness.

The Issue of Salt

Macrobiotic dietary recommendations include the moderate and regular use of salt and salt-based products. This idea runs counter to current trends warning that salt is to be avoided at all costs. This misconception has arisen in reaction to present dietary imbalances, and is another example of the macrobiotic principle that anything, in the extreme, will attract its opposite.

As a nation, we consume relatively large amounts of animal and dairy food. These have a high salt content. Cow's milk, for instance, contains as much as 1.6 grams of salt per liter. This is three times as much as human milk. Animal and dairy foods are also high in fat. The combination of excessive salt and excessive fat and protein is particularly harmful to health. Since these items are not easily broken down in the body, they tend to accumulate, leading to multiple health problems.

A second problem concerns the quality of salt we consume. Table salt is a highly processed item. Its minerals have been removed, although iodine is then returned to prevent *goiter*, an enlargement of the thyroid gland. Because necessary nutrients are removed, we often end up craving or using excessive amounts of salt, as the body signals nutritional deficiences by creating urges for certain foods.

Throughout history, cultures have recognized salt's importance. Salt was sacred to the ancient Aryans. The Greeks believed that bread (grains) and salt were gifts from the gods. The world "salt" comes from the Roman God of health. *Salus*. The Bible has a number of references to salt. In *Numbers* 18: 19 it says, "It is a covenant of salt for ever before the Lord unto thee and to thy seed with thee." The fifth century statesman Cassiodorus said it simply and perhaps best, "It may well be that some seek not gold, but there lives not a man who does not need salt."

Our body contains about three-and-a-half ounces of salt. This is maintained at a fairly constant level. The addition of salt during cooking helps ensure our mineral balance. Sea salt contains trace elements in small but necessary amounts. The proper use of sea salt strengthens and maintains our general health by keeping our blood quality slightly alkaline. It strengthens red and white blood cells, which in turn enhances our immune system. The balanced use of sea salt also strengthens all body organs and especially the kidneys and the heart.

Besides sea salt itself, there are a variety of salt-based products that are used regularly. Miso and tamari soy sauce are fermented products made with sea salt, grains, and beans. Sea vegetables also contain minerals, as do many traditionally prepared pickles and condiments. These help to satisfy our taste and nutritional need for salt.

There are also different variations of the salt taste that subtly influence various organs and systems in the body. We consume a sour/pungent salt in the form of sauerkraut and umeboshi plum, and a bitter salt in the form of sea vegetable powders.

A diet of grains, beans, and vegetables is generally low in sodium. The use of salt in cooking helps make foods more tasty. And, as anyone who has eaten a macrobiotic meal can testify, in the hands of a skilled cooked, salt is a flavor-enhancer, making food most delicious.

The Importance of Cooking

Our eating habits over the past sixty years have carried us from a naturally balanced diet that maintained lifetime health to one of increasing extremes. Along with this trend has been the loss of cooking skills. Many of us do not really know how to cook. Yes, we can heat things up in a microwave oven, or put a tin-foil dinner into the oven, but this is not cooking. The skillful and colorful blending of ingredients, and the use of flame or fire, is really an art, perhaps the highest art. By our selection and preparation of food, we either become healthy and happy, or sick and miserable. With proper cooking we not only control our own health, but through the quality of our reproductive cells, we influence the well-being of generations yet to be born.

In the macrobiotic kitchen, we use common, everyday foods, in their natural and unprocessed form. This requires know-how in preparation. How to skillfully blend these into delicious, attractive, and healthful meals that we can enjoy day after day is most important. This means that we may have to learn the art of cooking. The best way to do this is with an experienced macrobiotic cook. If this is not possible, there are a variety of excellent cookbooks that can be of help. The companion volume in the *Macrobiotic Food and Cooking*

Series contains complete directions for all foods recommended in this book. In addition, it has a wealth of general information for beginning macrobiotic cooks.

A second important consideration in regard to cooking is the type of flame we use. Throughout history fire has been a source of mystery, inspiration, and awe. Many cultures considered fire to be sacred, the connection between this world and the next. During the height of the Roman empire, each household had a family fire, which was thought to contain the family's guiding spirit. It was most important to keep this flame burning or face the loss of this spiritual guidance.

Cooking has had an enormous impact on biological evolution. Fire is a major factor setting us apart from the rest of the animal kingdom. Eating uncooked foods leaves the rest of the animal kingdom at the mercy of the environment. During the warmer months when food is plentiful, animals tend to be most active. As the weather cools and vegetation dies, food supplies grow scarce. Some animals then migrate to warmer climates, to await the return of spring. Others hibernate during the cold, dark months to reawaken in spring and begin foraging for food. Human beings, however, know the secret of fire and use it not only for external heat, but also to cook food and take fire inside their bodies. By doing this we maintain bodily heat, strength, nutrition, and activity throughout the year.

The use of fire makes our food yang. It gives active energy to foods, resulting in the fusion of elements. A mixture of uncooked brown rice, fresh spring water, and a pinch of sea salt, would not be very appetizing. But, with the addition of fire, these elements fuse, producing a delicious, energizing dish. This fusion is an example of fire's yangizing effect.

Cooking with fire is orderly. The heat from fire moves from the outside towards the inside. This movement from periphery to center represents a yang or contracting spiralic movement. This characteristic has an important impact not only on the nutritional aspects of food, but on its energy and vitality as well.

The use of fire for cooking has been decreasing steadily in recent decades. Electricity is being used more and more often. Electricity is a flow of electrons. Heat is generated from this current, and food is thus "cooked." But the nature of fire from combustion and electrically generated heat are very different. Electricity follows the path of least resistance. Its energy movement and effect differs from the orderly movement and effect of the movement of a flame's heat from periphery to center.

The newest innovation of modern technology is the microwave oven. Approximately 60 percent of American homes now have this

110

device. A microwave oven does not cook food in the true sense of the word—it radiates it. Microwaves move in a random fashion. As they penetrate a food item they begin to cause random collisions of its molecules. These collisions cause friction and heat, which result in the warming of food from the inside out. This reflects energy movement from the center to the periphery, a yin (expanding) spiral which is opposite to the yang (contracting) spiral of fire.

The effect of microwave cooking is to neutralize the central, yang elements of food and to expand the more yin peripheral elements. As a result, food loses its power to nourish and strengthen us. In this sense, microwave ovens do not cook foods, they radiate and destroy them. In the long run, eating such foods can only weaken our health.

Fire, from either wood or gas, is the most effective method to accomplish our goal of continued or renewed health. It is strongly recommended that everyone, not just those who are in the process of regaining their health, avoid microwave and electric cooking devices.

Lifestyle Suggestions

The following are a list of way of life suggestions that in cooperation with a macrobiotic way of eating provide a total plan of health regeneration.

- Live each day happily without being preoccupied with your health, and try to keep mentally and physically active.
- View everything and everyone you meet with gratitude, particularly offering thanks before and after every meal.
- Please chew your food very well, at least 50 times per mouthful or until it becomes a liquid.
- It is best to retire before midnight and get up early every morning.
- It is best to avoid wearing synthetic or woolen clothing directly on the skin. As much as possible, wear cotton, especially for undergarments. Avoid excessive metallic accessories on the fingers, wrists, or neck. Keep such ornaments simple and graceful.
- If your strength permits, go outdoors in simple clothing. Walk on the grass, beach, or soil up to one-half hour every day. Keep your home in good order, from the kitchen, bathroom, bedroom, and living room, to every corner of the house.
- Initiate and maintain an active correspondence, extending your best wishes to parents, children, brothers and sisters, teachers and friends.
- Avoid taking long hot baths or showers unless you have been consuming too much salt or animal food.

- Scrub your entire body with a hot damp towel until the skin becomes red every morning or every night before retiring. If that is not possible, at least scrub your hands, feet, fingers, and toes.
- Avoid chemically perfumed cosmetics. For care of teeth, brush with natural preparations or sea salt.
- If your condition permits, exercise regularly as part of daily life, including activities like scrubbing floors, cleaning windows, and washing clothes. You may also participate in exercise programs such as yoga, martial arts, dance, or sports.
- Avoid using electric cooking devices (ovens and ranges) or microwave ovens. Convert to gas or wood-stove cooking at the earliest opportunity.
- It is best to minimize the use of color television and computer display units.
- Include some large green plants in your house to freshen and enrich the oxygen content of the air of your home.

Each of these suggestions, when put into practice, will have a positive influence on our well-being. However, several of them merit special attention for reproductive disorders and infertility.

Chewing Well.   The importance of chewing our foods well cannot be stressed enough. Thorough chewing allows for easier digestion and more complete absorption. Our bodies make healthy new cells from this digested food and chewing is another tool to be used for our overall health.

An added benefit of chewing is that it releases more of the taste of food. This is especially true of complex carbohydrates, of which whole grains are an example. The more we chew them, the sweeter they become. Please make a conscious effort to chew your food well.

Scrubbing the Whole Body.   Scrubbing the whole body stimulates the circulation of blood, lymph, and energy. It helps break down any stagnation or accumulation that may have developed from past dietary and lifestyle imbalances. Scrubbing in the morning makes one feel energized and active, whereas scrubbing at night will enable one to relax and sleep better.

Cooking.   Since eating is basic to our survival, how we cook our food becomes very important. Cooking on either gas or wood is recommended because it strengthens and fully energizes what we cook on it. If you have either an electric range or microwave oven, an immediate change can be made by using a portable two- or three-burner gas stove until a full-sized gas stove can be purchased or an arrangement made for daily access to one.

Helping Our Mind and Emotions ────────────────

Accompanying the biological problems of reproductive disorders and infertility are the mental and emotional aspects. Their impact, in the form of worry, guilt, anxiety, self-doubt, depression, anger, and confusion, can be as devastating as their physical counterparts. The adoption of proper diet and lifestyle is the essential step for relief. Once this is accomplished, mental and emotional troubles will diminish and eventually dissolve. This renewal takes place along with, and as part of, our biological recovery.

This process of physical and mental renewal is not, however, like the apparently straight path of a rocket ship taking off. Overall, we are going in the direction of renewed health, but during this journey we experience fluctuations. To help ourselves through these times of ups and downs, there are many, many tools available to us. An excellent resource book the reader may wish to consult is the author's *Book of Dō-In: Exercise for Physical and Spiritual Development.* This book provides a variety of practices that can be used daily to improve the health and vitality of our complete self—physical, emotional, and spiritual. Following is a brief description of some practices the reader can use.

Daily Order and Activity: By keeping our immediate surroundings clean and orderly we are creating an environment that fosters a bright and optimistic outlook. This is especially important in our home and workplace, where we spend the majority of our time. It is best to permit the free flow of fresh air and sunlight, rather than keeping the atmosphere dark and stale. This is also true for rooms where we sleep. During the day, windows and blinds should be opened to let in fresh air and sunshine so that when we return there to sleep, the room's energy has been refreshed. When weather permits, a window can be kept slightly open at night to provide fresh air circulation. Assorted green plants can be kept nearby.

Physical Activity: Some type of comfortable daily activity is desirable to stimulate circulation and the discharge of toxins. Physical activity brightens our mental and emotional states and enhances the feeling that we are capable of helping ourselves. Rhythmic activities such as Do-In, yoga, t'ai ch'i dance, or other sports are fine. The purpose is to stimulate circulation rather than to exhaust ourselves.

Contact with Nature: The flow of Heaven's and Earth's force is continuous. By being outside some time every day, we receive the benefit of these fully charging our bodies. A 20- to 30-minute daily walk in a more natural surrounding is an almost fool-proof antedote to mental and emotional upsets.

Prayer: Daily prayer provides the opportunity to give thanks for our wonderful potential to improve our health. Any kind of prayer, including self-composed ones, is fine.

Self-reflection: By reflecting on our past behavior we realize that we have created our own problems. We acknowledge that we must change. This is not guilt. It is reflection that leads to understanding, insight, and self-realization. By practicing this we will realize that we have the freedom to change sickness and misery into health and happiness.

Singing and Chanting: Singing vibrates our whole body and releases energy in the form of sound vibrations. This not only affects our physical body, but also lifts our mental and emotional energy. Many of us are already using this unconsciously when we sing along with music from the radio in the car or at home. Every major spiritual belief has some type of chanting or repetition of a prayer or sound, whereby individuals can change the vibration of their whole being.

The energy effect of chanting certain sounds is very powerful. It influences the vibration of the whole body, and specific sounds influence specific areas and organs of the body. Daily we are intuitively using sound. Examples include the way we alter our voice when we speak to another in order to obtain a certain reaction; the sound of another person's voice and the effect it has on us; or the sounds that come from the immediate environment and how we react to them. We can use this power to help ourselves. In the *Book of Dō-In*, mentioned above, various chants are explained. Readers are encouraged to refer to this and other sections of the book for helpful suggestions.

Meditation: By sitting erect in a comfortable position and quieting our minds we can have an enormous influence over our body. This posture harmonizes all our biological processes and permits a freer flow of Heaven's and Earth's force through us. Our mental and emotional states become smooth and peaceful, diminishing any wild thoughts or self-conscious chatter in our heads. This practice can be done by itself or coupled with sound to initially harmonize our energy and permit more effective practice.

Breathing Exercise: Controlling our breath is another method to influence our body's total energy. Slow, smooth breathing with a slightly longer exhalation than inhalation can be practiced daily. The gentle evenness of this type of breathing harmonizes the flow of Heaven's and Earth's force through our body, resulting in a very peaceful state.

Mental Imagery: The creation of mental images or pictures is a very powerful method to influence ourselves. The variety of images we can create is endless. The effect of this imaging is that our body begins to align itself or become this image. As we eat well and continue to practice, our images become stronger and more powerful.

Social Contact: After we begin the practice of macrobiotics, it is important not to try to practice alone. If at all possible, initiate and maintain contact with other macrobiotic people. With them we can exchange ideas and experiences and continue learning. This helps to dispel the feeling that one is the only person in the world to experience certain problems. Many others have also been through similar experiences and their stories and example can be a great help.

All of these methods and others are available to help us in our return journey to health. In the Berkshire Mountains in western Massachusetts I have established a center to teach these various methods in what I call *Spiritual Seminars*. This training is available to anyone who is interested and wishes to deepen their understanding and practical application of these practices.

Calming the Mind and Emotions

The foods that can cause infertility and reproductive disorders can also create other problems in our body. One particularly widespread condition can have a devasting impact on our well-being.

A diet of eggs, chicken, and dairy products can have a strong influence on the pancreas. The function of the pancreas is to secrete both digestive enzymes and the complementary/antagonistic hormones, insulin and glucagon, or anti-insulin.

Insulin brings blood-sugar levels down, resulting in a more yang condition. Glucagon has an opposite effect. It stimulates the release of sugar from the liver and muscles, creating a more yin condition. These two functions have a huge influence on the body's energy level. With a balanced dietary practice, the pancreas works well, and our energy level is steady. However, when the pancreatic functions are disrupted, we can experience a bewildering array of physical, mental, and emotional symptoms. This is especially true if the secretion of glucagon is blocked.

Glucagon is more yin, so a diet of chicken and eggs, which are yang, can easily neutralize it. The fat in dairy food can coat the pancreas and block the secretion of this hormone. This results in falling energy levels, and in reaction, produces an intense craving for simple sugars, and often, a huge appetite.

A drop in our energy level is experienced in co-ordination with environmental energies. This tends to occur in the afternoon, especially between the hours from 2 P.M. to 5 P.M. At this time we can experience weakness ranging from mild fatigue to exhaustion. We may want to rest, and if this condition is extreme, we may feel that we could lay down wherever we happen to be and go immediately to sleep. Because the sugar level is low, the body is conserving energy and making balance by forcing us to rest.

Accompanying this biological reaction are a number of mental and emotional states. We can feel irritable, grumpy, tense, confused, forgetful, inattentive to what is going on around us, anxious, and worrisome. In extreme cases we become depressed, especially in the evening. As night progresses we can become fearful. We may not want to go out, instead seeking the support of a friend or spouse, perhaps actually clinging to them to help us through these feelings. We may awaken in the middle of the night with fear and anxiety and have difficulty getting back to sleep.

This spectrum of emotional and mental states is due to problems relating to our blood sugar level. We can correct this condition by following a balanced macrobiotic way of eating. In addition, there is a supplementary self-care practice we can use to ease these mental and emotional symptoms.

We begin by sitting straight in a chair with our hands together in prayer position about chest high. We breath in through our mouth, pulling the air up toward the center of our brain. Upon exhaling we chant the sound su, pronounced like the name Sue. We do this comfortably until our full exhalation is released. This can be repeated five times. Then our right palm is placed over the stomach region. This will send energy to the stomach, spleen, and pancreas region, and harmonize their functions. We keep our palm there about ten minutes. Our left arm can hang down or rest on our lap. The purpose is not to press our palm against this middle region but to have it lightly touching or a short distance away.

This practice can also be done lying on the back and placing the right palm over the stomach region. The left hand and arm is relaxed on the floor. After this is done for ten minutes, we can massage the stomach meridian to further regularize the energy of our stomach, spleen, and pancreas. We can begin to massage the stomach meridian below the knee, on the outside of the leg according to Figure 16.

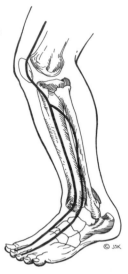

Fig. 16
The stomach meridian runs down the outside of the leg to the second and third toes. This can be massaged starting just below the knee down to the toes.

When there are pancreatic problems, the related meridian can be very tight. By giving a good massage, through pressing and releasing, we stimulate the free flow of energy through it. This can be done three to five times. The stomach meridian ends in two branches. One goes to the second toe, the other to the middle toe. Both toes can be pressed between the thumb and fingers and also pulled away from the foot at the same time. Do this ten times for each toe. The stomach meridian of the left leg and right leg can both be treated. This permits the discharge of excessive energy.

If someone is willing to help, they can massage the stomach meridian while the person lays on his or her back. Then they can pull on the toes. This allows the person who is receiving the treatment to relax more completely. The effect of this treatment is to relax the whole body by releasing energy. The mental and emotional state will become calm and peaceful. Through proper diet and lifestyle, and using this practice, we can effectively treat the mental and emotional symptoms of infertility and reproductive disorders.

6. Modifying the Standard Macro biotic Diet ■────────

Standard macrobiotic dietary guidelines provide the basis for maintaining vital physical and mental health. They are in line with current recommendations for disease prevention issued by major governmental and professional agencies. They easily satisfy the full range of nutritional needs while providing the flexibility to support the uniqueness of each individual.

Specific health problems often require initial modifications according to their cause. These adjustments are based on the particular yin or yang nature of the problem and allow an individual to comfortably and safely regain a balanced condition. This initial period usually lasts from two to three months, and should be made with the guidance of a qualified macrobiotic instructor.

The modified version of standard dietary guidelines can be practiced by individuals experiencing major illnesses that affect the reproductive system. For reproductive disorders that can lead to infertility, specific temporary adjustments to the modified version of the "standard diet" can be made. For those unfamiliar to the Unifying Principle of yin and yang, these temporary adjustments provide a necessary and clear pattern of eating that can be comfortably followed.

Even within these short-term dietary adjustments, however, the macrobiotic way of eating offers a balanced and varied selection of foods and cooking styles. Often, the biggest challenge individuals face is to make full use of the variety.

Below is an explanation of the modified version of standard macrobiotic dietary guidelines. After that, specific adjustments are given for particular reproductive problems that can lead to infertility.

Modified Standard Macrobiotic Diet ────────

Grains:
- Brown rice may be eaten daily. It is to be pressure-cooked with a pinch of unrefined white sea salt. Brown rice can also be cooked once a week in the following ways for variety:
  Brown Rice + Millet (20 percent to 30 percent)
  Brown Rice + Barley (20 percent to 30 percent)
  Brown Rice + Beans (10 percent to 15 percent)
  For breakfast, left-over brown rice or other

grain can be boiled 10 to 15 minutes to make a softer, morning cereal dish.
- Secondary grains such as millet, barley, and corn on the cob can be eaten. Corn on the cob can be eaten 2 to 3 times per week during the summer months.
- Sourdough bread (unyeasted) can be taken 2 to 3 times per week. It can be steamed and eaten with soup.
- Noodles such as udon (whole wheat) or soba (buckwheat) and other pasta can be taken 2 to 3 times per week in a hot broth.
- For better health it is best to temporarily avoid all other baked-flour products such as crackers, cookies, chips, muffins, rolls, bread, and so on.

Soup:
- Two cups of soup may be taken per day.
- One cup of mugi (barley) miso soup is taken daily. This is prepared with wakame sea vegetable and a variety of vegetables.
- For a second soup, a selection can be made from the following list:
  Grain soup
  Bean soup
  Squash soup
  Vegetable soup
- Sea vegetables should be included in soups. Also, after either miso, tamari, or sea salt is added, the soup should be simmered to cook in these seasonings.

Vegetable Dishes:
- Nishime style: 2 to 3 times per week.
- Azuki-Squash-Kombu: 2 to 3 times per week.
- Daikon and green tops, or carrots and green tops, or turnip and green tops, or dandelion root and greens: 2 to 3 times per week.
- Dried Daikon and Kombu: 2 to 3 times per week.
- Boiled salad: daily
- Pressed salad: 3 to 4 times per week.
- Raw salad: 1 to 2 times per week in hotter summer months.
- Steamed greens: daily
- Sautéed vegetables: with oil 2 to 3 times per week. As a substitute for oil use water-sautéing.

- Kinpira: 2 to 3 times per week.
- Seitan, tempeh, tofu stew: 2 to 3 times per week.
- From this list of vegetable dishes a menu can be composed. Some things are taken on a daily basis, such as boiled salad, while others can be rotated according to the number of times per week.

Beans:
- "Regular use beans" such as azuki, black soybeans, lentils, and chick-peas can be taken 2 to 3 times per week.
- "Occasional use beans" such as kidney, split peas, turtle beans, and navy beans can be taken 2 to 3 times per month.
- Beans products such as tofu, dried tofu, tempeh, natto, and other bean products can be eaten 2 to 3 times per week.
- Practically speaking, beans are eaten, in small amounts, on a daily basis. Within an individual meal, two kinds of beans can be taken in separate dishes, such as tofu in the soup and azuki beans served as a side dish.

Sea Vegetables:
- One sheet of lightly toasted nori can be taken daily.
- Arame and hijiki can be eaten 2 to 3 times per week as a separate side dish.
- Wakame and kombu can be taken on a daily basis in soups, vegetable dishes, and cooked with beans.

Condiments:
- The following condiments can be used daily in a small volume:
  Gomashio
  Sea vegetable powder with roasted sesame seeds
  Tekka
  Umeboshi plums
- In addition, there are a variety of other condiments that can be used less often and according to taste. Examples include:
  Brown-rice vinegar
  Umeboshi vinegar
  Nori condiment
  Roasted sesame seeds or pumpkin seeds
  Shiso leaves

Shio Kombu
Green nori flakes

Pickles: • A small volume of pickles is eaten daily, usually after a meal. The following list provides a variety of selections:
Bran pickles
Brine pickles
Miso bean pickles
Miso pickles
Pressed pickles
Sauerkraut
Tamari soy sauce pickles
Takuan pickles

Fish: • White-meat fish can be taken 2 times per week. Some suggested selections are:
Carp
Cod
Flounder
Trout
Sole
Scrod
• Fish can be cooked in a variety of ways such as in soup, steamed, or boiled. As a garnish, grated daikon plus a few drops of tamari soy sauce can be added.

Fruit: • Fruit can be eaten about 2 times per week. These are northern fruits, not tropical fruits. Methods of preparation include cooking fruits with a pinch of sea salt, eating dried fruit, and fresh fruits with a pinch of sea salt. Fresh-fruit eating is best limited to melons and berries only during the hotter months of summer.

Nuts: • Twice per week a handful of nuts can be eaten. They can be lightly toasted with a pinch of sea salt or a few drops of tamari soy sauce. The following nuts can be eaten:
Almonds
Peanuts
Walnuts

Seeds: • Seeds can be taken about 2 to 3 times per week.

Pumpkin seeds
Sesame seeds
Squash seeds
Sunflower seeds
- Because sunflower seeds have the highest oil content, these are best taken only during the hotter months of summer.

Snacks:
- A snack is a small volume eaten between meals. It does not constitute a meal in and of itself. The following snacks can be eaten:
Leftovers
Noodles
Popcorn (without butter)
Puffed whole cereal grains
Rice balls
Rice cakes
Seeds
Sushi
Mochi
- Some of the above listed snacks are dry snacks such as rice cakes, popcorn, and puffed whole cereal grains. It is best to consume less of the dry snacks.

Sweet Vegetables:
- The following sweet vegetables can be used on a rotating daily basis to provide a rich, vegetable-quality sweet taste.
Onion
Cabbage
Carrot
Daikon
Parsnips
Squash
Pumpkin

Additional Sweets:
- The following can be taken, in small quantity, to satisfy additional sweet cravings.
Amazaké
Barley malt
Rice syrup
Chestnuts
Hot apple cider
Hot apple juice

Beverages:

- The following beverages can be used on a daily basis.
  Bancha twig tea
  Bancha stem tea
  Toasted barley tea
  Roasted brown rice tea
  Spring water
  Well water
- The following beverages can be taken occasionally, about 2 to 3 times per week.
  Grain coffee (100 percent grain, no beets, figs, or molasses)
  Dandelion tea
  Kombu tea
  Umeboshi tea
  Mu tea
  Carrot juice
- One should drink when thirsty. If not thirsty, there is no need to try and consume beverages according to a schedule. For health purposes, it is better to make carrot juice by grating carrots and squeezing out the juice instead of using an electric juicer.

Seasonings:

- Seasonings for everyday use include:
  Miso (mugi or barley miso)
  Tamari soy sauce
  Unrefined white sea salt (Do not use grey sea salt)
- In the use of miso, tamari soy sauce, and unrefined white sea salt, it is best to cook them after adding them to whatever we are preparing. After adding an appropriate amount of miso to broth, we simmer it 2 to 3 minutes. We do the same thing if we are using tamari soy sauce or sea salt.
- Seasonings which we can use on an occasional basis, 2 to 3 times per week include:
  Ginger
  Horseradish
  Mirin
  Rice vinegar
  Umeboshi plum
  Umeboshi paste

The above modifications in the Standard Macrobiotic Diet can be safely followed until general health and vitality improves. At that time, careful additions can be made to widen the scope of eating. A fuller, more comprehensive description of cooking and food selection is provided in the companion volume, *MFCS: Infertility and Reproductive Disorders.* Readers are encouraged to consult this book before attempting to begin a macrobiotic way of cooking and eating.

Dietary Adjustments ━━━━━━━━━━━━━━━━━━━━━━

The following section contains specific adjustments to the modified version of the Standard Macrobiotic Diet for the major reproductive health problems that can lead to infertility. When specific changes are not suggested, the modified version of the Standard Diet can be used.

For Low Sperm Count, No Sperm Count, or Poor Sperm Motility

Grains:
- Whole oats, if desired, should be taken only once every 10 days. For a time, avoid oatmeal (rolled oats).
- Sourdough bread can be eaten 2 times per week. It is to be steamed and taken with soup.
- Rice fried with oil is to be taken 1 time per week.

Soup:
- Sometimes Hatcho (soybean) miso can be used instead of mugi (barley) miso. There should be a good balance of all three types of vegetables— leafy green, round, and root.

Vegetable Dishes:
- Raw salad should generally be avoided except in summer, and then only when craved.
- Oil-sautéed vegetables can be eaten 2 to 3 times a week.
- It is best to use dried tofu instead of fresh tofu in the seitan, tempeh, tofu stew dish.

Beans:
- "Occasional use beans" should be used 1 to 2 times a month.
- The use of dried tofu is preferred over fresh tofu.

Sea Vegetables:
- Same as the modified Standard Diet.

Condiments:
- Gomashio can be made in a 16 to 1 proportion of sesame seeds to sea salt. If possible, good-

quality black sesame seeds can be used.
- One-half of an umeboshi plum can be eaten daily.
- Two good condiments to use are shio kombu and dried-fish condiment.

Pickles:
- Same as the modified Standard Diet.

Fish:
- White-meat fish can be eaten 2 times per week.
- Two additional fish dishes that are recommended are *Koi Koku* (carp soup) and salmon head cooked with soybeans.

Fruit:
- Minimize fruit for a time. Take only small amounts unless strongly craved, then take fruit cooked with a pinch of sea salt.
- In the hotter summer months some fresh fruit can be eaten, but again, only when craved. The best fresh fruit to eat is melons or berries with a pinch of sea salt.

Nuts:
- Do not eat nuts on a regular basis. Eat only sometimes in small amounts, such as a handful.

Seeds:
- Sunflower seeds are best eaten only in summer.

Snacks:
- Same as the modified Standard Diet.

Sweet Vegetables:
- Same as the modified Standard Diet.

Additional Sweets:
- These sweets are to be eaten only when additional sweet cravings are experienced. They are to be taken in small volume and can be prepared with kuzu or kanten.

Beverages:
- Same as modified Standard Diet.

Seasonings:
- Same as modified Standard Diet.

Way of Life Suggestions:
- It is very important to scrub the whole body with a cotton cloth morning and evening.
- No cooking on microwave or electric appliances.
- Chew your food well, until liquid.
- Do not eat 2 to 3 hours before bed.

Home Care:
- Ginger compress on the kidneys 2 times per week is optional. For directions consult the list at the end of this section.

Special Drinks: • A cup of *Ume-sho-kuzu* can be taken 1 to 2 times per week, for several weeks.

For Varicocele and Other Testicular Blockages

Grains:
- Use kombu, about a ½-inch piece, instead of sea salt in cooking grains.
- Do not eat oatmeal (rolled oats). Instead, use whole oats about once every ten days, if desired.
- Sourdough (unyeasted) bread can be eaten about once a week.
- If one has had an operation or biopsy in the past year, buckwheat groats and soba (buckwheat) noodles should be avoided. Instead, udon noodles may be eaten 2 to 3 times a week.

Soup:
- In mugi miso soup use daikon 3 times a week.
- The percentage of vegetables in soups should be about two-thirds leafy greens to one-third root vegetables.

Vegetable Dishes:
- Raw salad is best avoided. If strongly desired, it is best eaten only in the hotter summer months.
- In sautéing vegetables, it is best not to use oil; water-sauté instead. After one month oil can be used in sautéing 1 to 2 times per week.
- It is better to use dried tofu instead of fresh tofu in seitan, tempeh, tofu dish.

Beans:
- "Occasional use beans" should be avoided for one month, then eaten only 1 to 2 times a month.

Sea Vegetables:
- Same as the modified Standard Diet.

Condiments:
- Gomashio can be made in a 16 to 1 proportion of sesame seeds to sea salt.
- One-half of an umeboshi plum can be eaten daily for a few weeks.
- For a sour flavor, brown rice vinegar or umeboshi vinegar can be used on boiled salad or steamed greens.

Fish:
- If possible, no fish should be taken for up to one month. If fish is strongly craved, a 5-ounce serving can be taken occasionally. Use grated

daikon and a few drops of tamari soy sauce as a garnish.

Fruit:
- Minimize fruit for a time. If strong cravings arise, eat a small volume of fruit cooked with a pinch of sea salt.
- Raw fruit is to be avoided. If strongly craved, it is best taken with a pinch of sea salt, and only during the hotter summer months. The best raw fruit is berries or melons. Avoid tree fruit such as apples or peaches.

Nuts:
- It is best to avoid nuts for a while.

Seeds:
- It is best to avoid sunflower seeds.

Snacks:
- Do not overuse dry snacks such as rice cakes, puffed cereals, or popcorn.

Sweet Vegetables:
- Same as modified Standard Diet.

Additional Sweets:
- These sweets are to be used sparingly only when an additional sweet taste is strongly craved.

Beverages:
- Same as modified Standard Diet.

Seasonings:
- It is most important not to make food too salty. Seasoning tastes should be light and moderate.

Special Drinks:
- Take one cup of the following drink daily for ten days:

Grated carrot	(one-third cup)
Grated daikon	(one-third cup)
Nori sea vegetable	(one-half sheet)
Umeboshi plum	(one half plum)
Tamari soy sauce	(a few drops)

- Take 1 to 2 cups of Sweet Vegetable Broth daily for one month.
  For directions on preparing these drinks, consult the list at the end of this section.

Home Care:
- Every morning and evening scrub the whole body with a cotton cloth.
- Chew your food thoroughly, until it becomes liquid in the mouth.
- Do not eat 2 to 3 hours before bed.

For Male Hormonal Deficiency

Grains:	• Cook brown rice and azuki beans once a week. • It is best to take as little bread as possible, even sourdough (unyeasted) bread. If craved, take 1 or 2 slices per week, steamed and eaten with soup. • If one has had an operation or biopsy in the past year, avoid soba noodles or buckwheat.
Soup:	• Take two-thirds leafy greens to one-third root vegetables in soups.
Vegetable Dishes:	• Raw salad is best avoided. If strongly craved, take only in the hotter summer months. • Sautéed vegetables or rice can be made with oil once a week. The other times water-sauté. • Use dried tofu more often than fresh tofu in seitan, tempeh, tofu dish.
Beans:	• "Occasional use beans" should be taken only about once a month. • It is preferable to use dried tofu more often than fresh tofu.
Sea Vegetables:	• Same as modified Standard Diet.
Condiments:	• Gomashio can be made in a proportion of 16 parts sesame seeds to 1 part sea salt. Use good-quality black sesame seeds if available.
Pickles:	• Same as the modified Standard Diet.
Fish:	• A small 5-ounce serving of white-meat fish can be eaten once per week. This is best prepared in miso soup, steamed, or boiled.
Fruit:	• Eat fruit only when craved. Fruit cooked with a pinch of sea salt is best.
Nuts:	• It is best to avoid nuts for a time.
Seeds:	• Sunflower seeds are best eaten only in summer.
Snacks:	• Same as the modified Standard Diet.
Sweet Vegetables:	• Same as the modified Standard Diet.
Additional Sweets:	• These sweets are to be eaten only when craved and then in small amounts.

Beverages:	• Same as modified Standard Diet.
Seasonings:	• Same as modified Standard Diet.
Home Care:	• It is very important to scrub the body morning and evening with a cotton cloth. • Chew well, until your food is liquid. • Do not eat 2 to 3 hours before bed. • A ginger compress can be applied to the kidneys twice a week.
Special Drinks:	• One cup of ume-sho-kuzu can be taken twice a week for several weeks.

For Infections of the Genitourinary Tract

Grains:	• Brown rice cooked with azuki beans can be taken once per week. • Instead of sea salt, kombu can be used occasionally in cooking grains. • Oatmeal (rolled oats) should not be taken frequently. Whole oats can be eaten once about every ten days, if desired. • Sourdough (unyeasted) bread can be eaten 1 to 2 times a week, steamed and eaten with soup. • With noodles, it is best to take udon only 2 to 3 times per week.
Soup:	• Use more leafy green vegetables in soups than roots.
Vegetable Dishes:	• It is best to avoid raw salad for a while. • In sautéing vegetables, it is best to use water instead of oil for one month. After that, oil sautéing can be used 1 to 2 times a week.
Beans:	• "Occasional use beans" should be eaten only once a month.
Sea Vegetables:	• Same as modified Standard Diet.
Condiments:	• Gomashio can be made with a 16 to 1 proportion of sesame seeds to sea salt. • One-half of an umeboshi plum can be eaten daily.
Pickles:	• Same as modified Standard Diet.
Fish:	• The less fish the better. Eat only when craved,

not on a regular basis. The best ways to prepare fish are in soup, steamed, or boiled. The amount eaten is about a 5-ounce serving.

Fruit:
- For a time, fruit can be avoided. However, if craved, eat only fruit cooked with a pinch of sea salt. If fresh fruit is craved, eat melons or berries with a pinch of sea salt.

Nuts:
- It is best to avoid nuts for a while.

Seeds:
- It is better to avoid sunflower seeds. In the summer months a small volume of seeds can be eaten.

Sweet Vegetables:
- Same as modified Standard Diet.

Additional Sweets:
- Use these sweets only when craved. They may be cooked with kuzu or kanten (agar-agar) occasionally.

Beverages:
- Same as modified Standard Diet.

Seasonings:
- Same as the modified Standard Diet.

Home Care:
- Scrub the whole body morning and evening with a cotton cloth.
- Do not eat 2 to 3 hours before bed.
- Chew food thoroughly until it becomes liquid in the mouth.
- Wear cotton clothes, especially undergarments and other items touching the skin.

Special Drinks:
- Ume-sho-kuzu can be taken 2 times a week for a few weeks. For directions, consult the list at the end of this section.

For Endometriosis

Grains:
- Use a piece of kombu, about ½-inch square, per cup of grain. This is in place of sea salt.
- Sourdough (unyeasted) bread can be eaten about 1 to 2 times per week. Steam it and eat it with soup.

Soup:
- Take daikon in miso soup 3 times per week.
- Use more leafy greens than root vegetables in soups.

Vegetable Dishes:
- Take daikon and its tops, or carrot and its green tops, or turnip and its green tops, or dandelion root and dandelion greens 3 to 4 times per week.
- Do not eat raw salad for now.
- In sautéing, use water instead of oil for 1 month, then use oil about once a week.
- It is better to take dried tofu than fresh tofu in the seitan, tempeh, tofu dish.

Beans:
- Do not eat "occasional use beans" for 1 month.
- In bean products, use dried tofu instead of fresh.

Sea Vegetables:
- Same as the modified Standard Diet.

Condiments:
- Gomashio can be made in a 16 to 1 proportion of sesame seeds to sea salt. If available, use good-quality black sesame seeds.
- Take ½ of an umeboshi plum daily for a month or so.

Pickles:
- Same as the modified Standard Diet.

Fish:
- It is best to avoid fish for a time. However, if strongly craved, take a 5-ounce serving of white-meat fish only in soup, steamed, or boiled.

Fruit:
- If possible, no fruit should be eaten. However, if strongly craved, fruit cooked with a pinch of sea, take a small amount of salt or fresh fruit—melons and berries only—with a pinch of sea salt.

Nuts:
- It is better to avoid nuts for a while.

Seeds:
- No sunflower seeds should be eaten for a while.

Snacks:
- Same as the modified Standard Diet.

Sweet Vegetables:
- Same as the modified Standard Diet.

Additional Sweets:
- When an additional sweet taste is craved, eat only in small volume.

Beverages:
- Same as the modified Standard Diet.

Seasonings:
- Same as the modified Standard Diet.

Home Care:
- It is important to scrub the whole body daily, morning and evening.
- Chew each mouthful thoroughly, until liquid.
- Do not eat 2 to 3 hours before bed.

- If health permits, any physical activity that can be comfortably done is recommended.
- Do daikon hip bath and douche twice a week for 1 month. This is explained at the end of this section.

Special Drinks:
- Drink Sweet Vegetable Broth, 1 cup daily, for about 3 to 4 weeks.
- Every day for ten days, drink one cup of the following: grated carrot (one-third cup)
grated daikon (one-third cup)
nori (one-half sheet)
tamari soy sauce (a few drops)
- One cup of kombu tea can be taken 2 to 3 times a week.
Please consult the end of this section for directions on preparing these special drinks.

For Fibroid Tumors

Grains:
- Use a piece of kombu, about ½-inch square, instead of sea salt in cooking grains.
- Do not eat oatmeal (rolled oats). If desired, take whole oats about once every 2 weeks.
- It is best not to eat bread unless craved. Then sourdough (unyeasted) bread can be steamed and eaten with soup.
- Minimize the intake of soba noodles and kasha. Instead, have udon 2 to 3 times a week in soup.

Soup:
- In miso soup, take daikon 3 to 4 times a week.
- Use more leafy greens (two-thirds) to root vegetables (one-third).

Vegetable Dishes:
- Do not take raw salad.
- Water-sauté vegetables for the first month. Use oil for the second month about once per week.
- In kinpira, do not take oil, water-sauté instead. Do this for 1 month.
- In setain, tempeh, tofu stew dish, dried tofu is preferrable to fresh tofu.

Beans:
- Do not take "occasional use beans" for 1 month. Then, they can be taken twice per month.
- It is better to use dried tofu than fresh tofu.

Sea Vegetables:	● Same as the modified Standard Diet.
Condiments:	● Gomashio should be made in a 16 to 1 proportion of sesame seeds to sea salt. ● Umeboshi plum can be eaten 2 to 3 times a week. ● Shiso leaves can be used 2 to 3 times a week.
Pickles:	● Same as the modified Standard Diet.
Fish:	● It is best not to eat fish for an initial one-month period. If craved, take only white-meat fish in miso soup, steamed, or boiled. Garnish with grated daikon and tamari soy sauce. The amount of fish should be small, about a 5-ounce serving.
Fruit:	● If possible, no fruit should be taken for a while. If craved, cooked fruit can be taken in a small volume with a pinch of sea salt. ● If fresh fruit is craved, take only melons or berries and use a pinch of sea salt.
Nuts:	● Avoid nuts for the time being.
Seeds:	● Do not eat sunflower seeds for now. ● Other seeds eaten should be lightly roasted but no tamari soy sauce or sea salt should be added.
Snacks:	● Dry snacks such as rice cakes, popcorn, and puffed cereal grains should be eaten less often.
Sweet Vegetables:	● Same as the modified Standard Diet.
Additional Sweets:	● For sweet cravings, a small volume of these sweets can be taken. They are not to be taken on a regular basis.
Beverages:	● Same as the modified Standard Diet.
Seasonings:	● Same as the modified Standard Diet.
Home Care:	● Do the whole-body scrub twice daily, in the morning and evening. ● Chew foods thoroughly. ● Do not eat 2 to 3 hours before bed.
Special Drinks:	● For sweet cravings, Sweet Vegetable Broth can be taken. One and sometimes two cups can be taken per day. ● A heaping tablespoon of grated daikon with

a few drops of tamari soy sauce can be eaten once daily for 10 days.

- As a beverage, one cup of kombu tea can be taken 2 to 3 times per week.

Home Care:
- A daikon hip bath followed by a douche can be done 2 to 3 times a week for about 1 month.

Additional Drinks:
- The following drinks are also helpful for fibroid tumors:
    a. Leafy green vegetables boiled with a small piece of wakame or kombu sea vegetable for a few minutes. One cup can be taken daily for 2 to 3 weeks.
    b. Cook daikon and a small piece of kombu for 10 to 15 minutes, and drink the liquid. One-half to one cup can be taken every other day for 2 to 3 weeks.

Problems with Cervical Stenosis and Cervical Mucus

Grains:
- It is best to avoid bread. However, if craved, sourdough (unyeasted) bread can be steamed and eaten with soup.
- Do not eat oatmeal (rolled oats) for a while. Instead, whole oats can be eaten once every 10 days, if desired.
- Minimize the use of buckwheat (kasha) and soba noodles.

Soup:
- It is most important to use sea vegetables in soups.
- Vegetables that can be emphasized in soups are leafy greens and daikon. Of course other vegetables are to be used also but leafy greens can be used more often.

Vegetable Dishes:
- Avoid raw salad for now.
- The use of oil should be minimal. In sautéed vegetables, use oil once a week. Vegetables can be water-sautéed 2 to 3 times a week.
- In seitan, tempeh, tofu dish, it is best to use dried tofu.

Beans:
- The use of "occasional use beans" should be

minimal. At most, take 1 to 2 times a month.
- In using bean products, use dried tofu more often than fresh tofu.

Condiments:
- Gomashio should be made in a 16 to 1 proportion of sesame seeds to sea salt.
- Umeboshi plum can be taken 2 to 3 times a week.
- Two helpful condiments are dried shiso leaves and green nori flakes.

Pickles:
- Same as the modified Standard Diet.

Fish:
- It is best to avoid fish for a time. If craved, take a small volume of white-meat fish prepared in miso soup, steamed, or boiled. Grated daikon and a few drops of tamari soy sauce can be used as a garnish.

Fruit:
- Fruit should be eaten only when craved. Then, take fruit cooked with a pinch of sea salt.
- If fresh fruit is craved, especially in the hotter summer months, eat only melons or berries with a pinch of sea salt.

Nuts:
- Avoid nuts for now.

Seeds:
- For a while, avoid sunflower seeds.

Snacks:
- The use of dry snacks, such as popcorn, puffed cereals, and rice cakes, should be minimized.

Sweet Vegetables:
- Same as the modified Standard Diet.

Additional Sweets:
- Take only when craved and then only in small amounts.

Beverages:
- Same as the modified Standard Diet.

Seasonings:
- Same as the modified Standard Diet.

Home Care:
- Scrub the whole body every morning and evening.
- Do not eat 2 to 3 hours before bed.
- Chew food thoroughly until liquid.
- Do daikon hip bath and douche twice a week for several weeks.

Special Drinks:
- Boil leafy green vegetables with a small piece of wakame or kombu for a few minutes. Drink 1 cup of the cooking liquid daily for 10 days. Then take 1 to 2 times a week for 1 month.

For Scarring and Adhesions in the Fallopian Tubes

Grains:
- If bread is craved, take sourdough (unyeasted) bread steamed and eaten with soup.
- Minimize buckwheat (kasha) and soba noodles.

Soup:
- Same as the modified Standard Diet.

Vegetable Dishes:
- Do not eat raw salad for 1 to 2 months.
- Use oil to sauté vegetables once a week and water-sauté twice a week. This can be followed for one or two months, before increasing the use of oil.
- Use dried tofu instead of fresh tofu in the seitan, tempeh, tofu dish.

Beans:
- "Occasional use beans" can be eaten 1 to 2 times a month.
- Among bean products, dried tofu is preferred over fresh tofu.
- Same as the modified Standard Diet.

Condiments:
- Gomashio can be made in a 16 to 1 proportion of sesame seeds to sea salt.
- Umeboshi plums can be used 2 to 3 times a week.
- Shiso leaves are helpful and can be used 2 to 3 times per week.

Pickles:
- Same as the modified Standard Diet.

Fish:
- Eat as little fish as possible. If craved, take a small portion of white-meat fish once a week either in soup, steamed, or boiled. Grated daikon and a few drops of tamari soy sauce can be used as a garnish.

Fruit:
- Take fruit occasionally when craved, not on a weekly schedule. Have only fruit cooked with a pinch of sea salt.
- If fresh fruit is craved during the summer, eat small amounts of melons or berries with a small pinch of sea salt.

Nuts:
- Do not eat nuts for a while.

Seeds:
- Do not eat sunflower seeds for a while.

Sweet Vegetables: ● Same as the modified Standard Diet.

Additional Sweets: ● When an extra sweet is craved, use these sweetners in small volume.

Beverages: ● Same as the modified Standard Diet.

Seasonings: ● Same as the modified Standard Diet.

Home Care:
● Scrub the whole body daily, morning and evening.
● Chew each mouthful thoroughly, until liquid.
● Do not eat 2 to 3 hours before bed.
● A dried daikon leaves hip bath and douche may be used twice a week for about 1 month.

Special Drinks:
● For sweet cravings, take one cup of Sweet Vegetable Broth daily. This can be one cup daily.
● A drink made from grated carrot, grated daikon, ½ sheet of nori, and a few drops of tamari soy sauce can be taken, one cup daily for 10 days. Then, take 1 to 2 times a week for about 1 month.
● Green leafy vegetables boiled with a small piece of wakame or kombu can be taken several times a week for a few weeks. The amount taken is 1 cup each time.

For Failure to Ovulate

Grains:
● Use a little more liquid in cooking grains.
● Minimize the intake of oatmeal (rolled oats). Whole oats can be eaten once every 2 weeks.
● Sourdough (unyeasted) bread can be taken when craved. This can be steamed and eaten with soup.
● Do not take soba noodles, use udon 2 to 3 times a week.

Soup: ● Use more leafy greens (two-thirds) to root vegetables (one-third).

Vegetable Dishes:
● Raw salad should be taken only when craved, but not on a regular basis.
● Sautéed vegetables can be made with oil once a week. Water-sautéed vegetables may be taken a few times per week.
● It is best to use dried tofu instead of fresh tofu in the seitan, tempeh, tofu dish.

Beans:	• "Occasional use beans" can be taken 1 to 2 times a month.
Sea Vegetables:	• Same as the modified Standard Diet.
Condiments:	• Gomashio can be made in a 16 to 1 proportion of sesame seeds to sea salt. • Umeboshi plum can be taken 2 to 3 times per week.
Pickles:	• Same as the modified Standard Diet.
Fish:	• Eat fish only when craved, not on a weekly or regular basis. A smaller volume of white-meat fish in soup, steamed, or boiled can be eaten.
Fruit:	• Eat fruit only when craved, not regularly. Take fruit cooked with a pinch of sea salt. • If fresh fruit is craved in summer, eat only melons or berries with a pinch of sea salt.
Seeds:	• No sunflower seeds should be eaten for a while.
Sweet Vegetables:	• Same as the modified Standard Diet.
Additional Sweets:	• Use these sweets for additional sweet cravings and take in small volume.
Beverages:	• A ½ cup of carrot or celery juice may be taken 2 to 3 times a week.
Seasonings:	• Same as the modified Standard Diet.
Home Care:	• Scrub the body daily, morning and evening. • Chew food well, until if becomes liquid. • Do not eat 2 to 3 hours before bed. • It is helpful to have green plants in your immediate environment.
Special Drinks:	• Take 1 to 2 cups of Sweet Vegetable Broth daily for 2 to 3 weeks. • Boil leafy greens 2 to 3 minutes and drink one cup of the cooking liquid daily for a few weeks.

For Pelvic Inflammatory Disease

Grains:	• It is best not to eat bread for a while. However, if craved, sourdough (unyeasted) bread can be steamed and eaten with soup.

138

- It is best to avoid oatmeal (rolled oats) for a while. Instead, whole oats can be eaten once every 10 days if desired.
- Minimize the use of buckwheat (kasha) and soba noodles.

Soup: • Same as modified Standard Diet.

Vegetable Dishes: • Avoid raw salad.
- For 1 month do not use oil in sautéing vegetables. During the second month, oil can be used once a week. During the third month, oil can be used twice a week. During this time it is fine to water-sauté vegetables 2 to 3 times per week.
- Dried tofu is preferable to fresh tofu in seitan, tempeh, tofu dish.

Beans: • The use of "occasional use beans" should be minimized. This means about 1 to 2 times a month.
- Among bean products, emphasize dried tofu over fresh tofu.

Sea Vegetables: • Same as the modified Standard Diet.

Condiments: • Gomashio can be made in a 16 to 1 proportion of sesame seeds to sea salt.
- Umeboshi plum can be taken 2 to 3 times per week.

Pickles: • Avoid ginger pickles for now.

Fish: • If experiencing pain, avoid fish until it diminishes. However, if craved, a small volume of white-meat fish can be eaten either in soup, steamed, or boiled.

Fruit: • It is best to avoid fruit. However, if craved, take a small volume of fruit cooked with a pinch of sea salt.
- Fresh fruit is best avoided. However, if craved during the hotter summer months, eat small amounts of melons or berries with a pinch of sea salt.

Nuts: • Avoid for now.

Seeds: • Do not eat sunflower seeds for now.

	• Other seeds may be lightly roasted, but do not add tamari or sea salt.
Snacks:	• Use less of the dry snacks such as popcorn, puffed cereals, and rice cakes.
Sweet Vegetables:	• Same as the modified Standard Diet.
Additional Sweets:	• Use these sweets in small volume only when an extra sweet taste is craved.
Beverages:	• Same as the modified Standard Diet.
Seasonings:	• Do not use ginger or horseradish for a while.
Home Care:	• Scrub the whole body daily, morning and evening. • Do not eat 2 to 3 hours before bed. • Chew each mouthful until liquid.
Special Drinks:	• Ume-sho-kuzu can be taken 2 to 3 times a month.

For Sexually Transmitted Diseases

Grains:	• Grains can be cooked either with a pinch of sea salt, or a ½-inch square of kombu, per cup of rice.
Soup:	• Hatcho (soybean) miso can be used sometimes in place of mugi (barley) miso.
Vegetable Dishes:	• Raw salad should be minimized. Take only when craved. • Vegetables can be sautéed in water instead of oil for 1 month. The second month, oil can be used once a week. During the third month, oil can be used twice a week.
Beans:	• "Occasional use beans" can be taken 2 to 3 times a month. • Dried tofu is to be used more often than fresh tofu. • Same as the modified Standard Diet.
Condiments:	• Gomashio can be made with a 16 to 1 proportion of sesame seeds to sea salt. • Umeboshi plum can be taken 2 to 3 times a week.
Pickles:	• Same as the modified Standard Diet.
Fish:	• When craved, white-meat fish can be eaten in

miso soup, steamed, or boiled. Garnish with grated daikon and a few drops of tamari soy sauce.

Fruit:
- It is best to take no fruit for a while. However, if craved, a small volume of fruit cooked with a pinch of sea salt is best.
- If fresh fruit is craved, especially during the hotter summer months, take only a small volume of melons or berries.

Nuts:
- Avoid for a while.

Seeds:
- Generally, sunflower seeds are to be minimized. In the hotter summer months they may be eaten in small quantities.
- Other seeds, such as pumpkin or sesame, can be lightly toasted, but without sea salt or tamari soy sauce added.

Snacks:
- Same as the modified Standard Diet.

Sweet Vegetables:
- Same as the modified Standard Diet.

Additional Sweets:
- Use these sweets only when an extra sweet taste is craved and eat only a small volume.

Beverages:
- Carrot juice may be taken, about $\frac{1}{2}$ to 1 cup, 2 times a week. For health reasons, it is best not to make carrot juice with an electric blender or juicer. Instead, carrots can be grated and then the juice squeezed out.

Seasonings:
- The use of ginger should be minimized.

Home Care:
- It is important to chew very well.
- Scrub the whole body daily, morning and evening, to stimulate circulation.

Special Drinks:
- For sweet cravings, take 1 cup of Sweet Vegetable Broth 2 to 3 times a week.
- Ume-sho-kuzu can be taken once or twice a week for 1 to 2 months.

A Note of Caution

Individuals who have undergone an operative procedure within the past year should avoid buckwheat noodles and kasha (whole-grain buckwheat). Buckwheat has a tightening effect on the body which may slow down the healing process.

For the same reason, pay special attention to the use of sea salt and the salt-based products including miso, tamari soy sauce, and the various macrobiotic condiments. These seasonings, when properly used, bring out the natural flavor of our foods. However, if used in excess, foods will simply taste salty, and our condition could become imbalanced.

Many of us have grown accustom to the idea that more is better. This outlook is a dominant theme in modern society. When extended to the link between food and health it appears as the concept that if a little of some item helps, then two, four, or even ten times as much will help that much more. This type of thinking has led to many of the problems that we, as individuals and as a society, face today. Remember, our goal is balance.

Final Recommendations

The preceding recommendations are not meant to be followed for an extended period of time. They are temporary suggestions designed to establish the foundation of health during the initial period of macrobiotic practice. When this is achieved, one's dietary plan should be broadened to include a wider variety of foods and cooking styles within the Standard Macrobiotic Diet.

This process of enlarging the scope of one's diet continues with the gradual improvement of health. Within a relatively short time, an individual should be able to enjoy the full range of the Standard Macrobiotic Diet. At this point our emphasis shifts to one of maintaining health for a lifetime.

As our understanding and application of the macrobiotic principles develops, we will be able to eat freely, according to our goals and aspirations. The practice of macrobiotics frees us from biological, mental, and emotional problems, and allows us to develop our humanity to its infinite possibilities.

During the period of transition from sickness to health, it is most helpful to seek the guidance of both a qualified macrobiotic instructor and a cook. A qualified cook can teach us the skills needed to properly prepare macrobiotic meals that are suited to our specific condition and needs. A qualified instructor can answer questions, and educate us concerning the macrobiotic approach to our particular problem. He or she can also suggest specific adjustments to balance our changing condition. With these factors on our side, we are giving ourselves the best opportunity to regain our health.

7. Personal Experiences ━━━━━

Included in this chapter are personal stories of individuals who, when faced with serious reproductive disorders, chose to begin the practice of macrobiotics. Through lifestyle and dietary adjustments they were able to change their reproductive problems from sickness to health. For each of these stores there are thousands of others, each representing individuals who have successfully made the same choice.

These case histories are personal profiles of courage. They are provided to inspire and encourage others who may be experiencing reproductive disorders. Each points the way to a life of health and happiness.

Endometriosis: Sherrie Seatz ━━━━━━━━━━━━━

In the fall of 1983, I started having symptoms that made me very uneasy. My mother had recently died of ovarian cancer and I saw myself with some of her symptoms, plus a few of my own.

My doctor told me to wait several months and if the symptoms continued, he would do a laparoscopy. Because of the emotional trauma I had recently experienced with my mother's illness and death, he felt that the problem could be in my mind. But I knew it was more than that.

My period was coming every twenty-one days with a flow of blood which lasted ten days. I was weak and rundown. I could fix dinner for my family, but then I would be ready for bed. I was experiencing pain that would sometimes double me over, forcing me to lie down until it passed. My abdominal area was also very sore.

On the first of December my doctor did a laparoscopy and was surprised by what he found—widespread endometriosis. My bowels were bound down with lesions and he wasn't sure about my intestines. He said I was damned if I had surgery and damned if I didn't. If I had the usual hysterectomy, he might have to do bowel surgery, and the removal of part of my intestines was a possibility. He said I might be worse off after the surgery. There was a drug that could be tried, but he cautioned that the side effects were often worse than the disease. He sent me home to live with the pain.

In January 1984 I bought a book on the macrobiotic approach to cancer, and it had a section on endometriosis. I felt that this was the answer to my problem, so I phoned the East West Foundation for more information.

Within four or five days after beginning macrobiotic dietary suggestions, I started to feel a new flow of life that had long been gone. Ten days after I began, my period started. It lasted only eight days (it had shortened by two days already) and I had a much more normal blood flow. I have not had any pain at all since beginning the macrobiotic approach.

Each month I got stronger, and all things seemed more normal and balanced. It took me nearly two years to completely eliminate my disease, but it was a wonderful two years. Along with the other improvements, I found that my hypoglycemia was diminishing, I lost two warts from my foot, and the arches in my feet were strengthened to the point that I no longer needed to wear orthodiscs in my shoes. I am grateful to macrobiotics for having changed my life, and for making each day fuller, richer, and positive.

Uterine Carcinoma: Elaine Nussbaum

In April 1980 I had a diagnostic procedure done to determine the cause of the excessive and prolonged menstrual bleeding I was experiencing. The doctor discovered a malignant tumor—a carcinosarcoma in the connective tissue on the wall of the uterus. I was given twenty radiation treatments, a radium implant, hormone medication, and both oral and intravenous chemotherapy. In August 1980 the doctor performed a radical hysterectomy and a *bilateral salpingo oophorectomy*—the removal of my ovaries. I continued to take chemotherapy.

In May 1982 I started having pain in the lower back, and despite medication it got progressively worse. I could neither sit nor lie down. In August, after a few days of standing up day and night, sleeping only on my husband's shoulder in a standing position, I went to an orthopedist. He confirmed a compression fracture and noted also that my vertebrae were partially collapsed. In order to prevent a total collapse of the vertebrae, I was put into a brace which extended from above the chest to the pelvic area and around the back.

The pain got worse and spread to my legs. I could no longer stand. My husband put me in a reclining chair and gave me strong pain-killers around the clock. Nothing stopped the pain.

In September I was carried to the hospital for more X-rays and scans. In addition to the compression fracture and the partially collapsed vertebrae, these pictures showed cancer on the lumbar spine, cancer on the thoracic spine and multiple metastatic deposits on both lungs.

I was given radiation again (a series of five treatments), then chemotherapy, then five more radiation treatments, then more chemotherapy. The usual program was ten rounds of chemotherapy, given at three to four week intervals. I was tired, weak, nauseous, and in pain.

In January 1983, after four cycles of chemotherapy, X-rays and scans were taken again. The tests showed that there was increased activity and progression of the cancer in the spine, and unchanged metastatic cancer in both lungs.

Toward the end of January, while opening the mail, I cut my finger on an envelope. Because my blood levels were so depressed from the chemotherapy, I was unable to fight the infection that set in. The paper-cut resulted in a ten-day hospital stay, including four blood transfusions, massive doses of intravenous antibiotics, and three days in isolation. It was decided that the chemotherapy I was getting was too strong; I would be put on something less toxic.

It was then that I realized conventional medicine was not going to work for me. I did some research on alternative methods, and I chose macrobiotics. Dr. Sattilaro's book, *Recalled by Life*, was was a great inspiration to me. I felt that if he could get well on such a program, I could too. In mid-February I started to wean myself from meat, dairy products, fruit and sugar, and to reduce to zero the thirty-eight pills I was taking daily. By the end of February, I was on a macrobiotic diet.

I began the diet in a hospital bed, a wheelchair, and a brace. In a short while, I started walking with the help of a walker, then with a cane. In April, a urinary problem that had plagued me for three years (a result of the original radiation) disappeared. In mid-May I took off the brace. On May 22, I walked up and down my block all by myself.

In June, I put away my wig; my hair, which had all fallen out from the chemotherapy, had grown back enough to be presentable. I returned the hospital bed. I started driving again. I resumed my studies towards my master's degree. In six months, I changed from a sick, depressed, pill-popping invalid to a happy, optimistic, and very grateful pain-free person.

The side effects of the diet have been mostly positive. I have had a few bouts with diarrhea, fatigue, flaky skin, and other non-debilitating forms of "discharge." On the positive side, I enjoy good health, good energy, and perfect bodily functions, such as appetite, sleep, elimination, and mental alertness. And I really enjoy the food— my whole family does too.

Although I take no treatment or medications, I continue to see my oncologist periodically for check-ups. She says that I am doing very well.

I attribute the reversal of my cancer solely to macrobiotics, and I hope that my story will be a source of hope and inspiration to others.

Dermoid Tumor: Audrey Isakson

In the spring of 1977, Audrey Isakson of Kennebunkport, Maine, began to have very frequent menstrual periods and considerable back pain. "My doctor advised me to get into the hospital immediately and have surgery," she recounted, after a large tumor was discovered on her right overy. "But I decided to first try to heal it myself through macrobiotics." She had just read Gloria Swanson's article in *East West Journal* and resolved to relieve her own uterine condition before submitting to surgery.

In August she attended the East West Foundation's summer program at Amherst College and in September visited Edward Esko, a macrobiotic consultant in Boston. In addition to dietary adjustments, he recommended that she apply a taro potato plaster over the afflicted region and take regular daikon hip baths. In a short time Audrey's back pain subsided, and her menstrual periods started to become normal again.

"I went to the doctor six weeks after I had first seen her, and she examined me," Audrey related. The orange-size growth was gone. "How can you explain that it went away?" she asked the doctor. "I can't," the physician responded. Audrey then told her about the nutritional approach she had tried. "I'm rather skeptical," the doctor told her. "I really don't believe those kinds of things. But it seems to have worked for you." A final medical checkup four months later confirmed that "my ovary had returned to its normal size."

Prostatitis: Rick Chaff

It has been so long now since my nightmarish two-year ordeal with a prostate problem ended; I'd almost forgotten how miserable I was. I first experienced the symptoms five years ago. It started with a dull pain and feeling of irritation in the rectal area. I also experienced difficult and incomplete urination and weak ejaculation during sex. The act of sex itself was an unsatisfying experience. I finally decided it was time to see a doctor.

The first doctor I went to diagnosed my condition as *prostatitis* (an infection in the prostate gland) and gave me a prescription for an antibiotic. When that antibiotic didn't work, he gave me a stronger one. I remember feeling some hope with these antibiotics because they did provide temporary relief. But they failed to heal the condition. Next I tried going to an herbalist, a homeopathic doctor, and then a vitamin therapist. I took nine tablets for a while, which also provided some temporary relief, but again the symptoms returned. During this time I was becoming more and more irritable. The constant awareness of my condition was creating a lot of stress in my life. I would always be wondering whether it was getting better or worse. I would be hopeful, then disappointed. With the failure of each new therapy, I felt more frustrated and helpless.

I again decided to seek the advice of a medical physician. This one told me the next step would be surgery. By that time I was almost open to the idea just to end the constant stress and pain I was living with. They my best friend, Marlene, who is now my wife, told me about macrobiotics. She had used macrobiotics successfully to treat an ulcer condition. At first I was against the idea. I developed a nasty disposition and was angry about the whole situation. I was through with trying new remedies and it took Marlene a long time to convince me to schedule a consultation. She told me that if I really wanted to find a cure I should try everything. I finally gave in and decided to give it a try, but I had big doubts that it would do any good.

I went to see Edward Esko at the East West Foundation in Brookline, Massachusetts. Marlene and I met with Esko at the Seventh Inn, at that time a popular macrobiotic restaurant in Boston. First he told me everything I shouldn't eat. The list was long. Then he began telling me about the foods I should go out and get.

When we left Esko, I had a feeling that I had already gained some control over my prostate problem. What he had told me somehow made sense. I went out and bought sea vegetables, umeboshi plums, miso, brown rice, and fresh vegetables. These were now my weapons to fight this disease.

In the first ten days of following the diet, I did indeed notice a change. It felt as if there was a dramatic release in my prostate gland, as if it were free to "breathe" again. I felt a warm glow around the whole area. I knew that inside, a healing process was taking place. By this time, I had a personal relationship with my prostate gland; I always knew how it was feeling.

It was difficult for me to stay on the diet at first because at that time I was traveling and playing in a rock band. I had to pack enough food to last a week at a time. I ate a lot of rice balls during that period. I would also bring along a large jar of miso soup with lots of vegetables since this was sometimes the only way I could get them. And I always had a ready supply of rice cakes and yinnie syrup. I became the odd member in the band because of my unusual diet. Eventually, the other members became supportive and even started trying some of my rice balls.

Although the beginning changes were dramatic, it took several more months before my prostate condition was completely cleared. But there were several other side effects that were unexpected benefits. It seemed like my circulation was better, my breathing more open and complete, and my thinking clearer. I think I may also have had an undiagnosed hypoglycemic condition because I always felt tired and sleepy. After about a month, these symptoms went away as well. I had more energy than I had had in a long time. My eyes and complexion also looked clearer, and my skin felt more pliable.

It was a long process altogether, but with the diet, Esko's additional supportive healing techniques (moxabustion and ginger compresses), and Marlene's continued support, I now feel that I am in a good state of health. When I started having satisfying sex with no pain in the prostate area, I knew I was healed.

Fibroid Tumor: Diane Silver

Since childhood Diane Silver had been ill constantly. She had pneumonia at age two, and her tonsils and adenoids were removed at the age of four. Beginning in 1957 she suffered from painful cystitis, and for the next fourteen years was treated every few months with sulfa. Pneumonia returned periodically for which she received antibiotics. Diane had a painful diaphragmatic hernia and had to sleep sitting up. She had premenstrual tension, edema, and severe menstrual cramps. In 1960 doctors removed a large mole growing on her forehead and told her she might have malignant melanoma. In 1969 a large fibroid tumor was surgically removed from her uterus. In 1971 a tumor was found in a lymph node on her neck, and she was diagnosed as having thyroid cancer.

During the next few years she had bumps on her back and breasts that turned out to be benign. The fibroid tumor, however, returned and her Pap tests were irregular. By the fall of 1975 her endocrinologists told Diane that she would have to take sulfa drugs for the rest of her life. Tests indicated the cancer had spread to her kidney.

One day in October 1975, while bedridden with pneumonia, Diane received a phone call that changed her life. It was from a young man named Alan Ginsberg, who introduced himself as a friend of a friend in New York. "When he heard my gasping and coughing he remarked, 'You sound sick,' " Diane said, recalling the conversation. "Yes, I have pneumonia, I rasped. 'What are you eating?' he said. Well, in all my thirty-eight years of life, no physician had ever asked what I was eating."

"I told Alan I was eating some cottage cheese, salad, lots of grapefruit and orange juice because I need fluids. He asked me if I had considered that there were nine to twelve grapefruits in the two or three glasses of juice I was having every day; that grapefruits grow in hot climates, 'That this is November and you're in Toronto in the winter and it's getting cold, and furthermore, cottage cheese and all dairy foods create mucus in the body, and you don't need any more mucus!' Was he some kind of nut, I wondered? Or was he making sense?"

Alan asked her if she had any whole grains in the house. She had only oatmeal, and he advised her to eat just oatmeal, with no milk or sugar on it, for several days, and he would call back. Diane was skeptical, but after a few days of just oatmeal she was out of bed, feeling better, and ready to listen to what Alan had to say. He called back, explained to her the principles of macrobiotics and sent her some books to read. After a few months on the diet, Diane was strong enough to begin to exercise and take short walks.

At the end of December 1975, I gave a lecture in Toronto and Diane came to see me. "Mr. Kushi reaffirmed for me everything Alan had said," she noted in reviewing her case. "He amazed me because he diagnosed all my conditions simply by looking at my face and feeling my arm. Mr. Kushi said that I was still cancerous and gave me a list of foods to eat and those to avoid."

When Diane subsequently gave up taking birth-control pills, she said, "My doctor assured me I would be back for a hysterectomy very shortly because the fibroid tumors would grow wildly without hormonal control. The following year at my regular check-up, he reported that they had disappeared—and that I was in better shape than I had been for years." Diane's Pap smear registered normal, her diaphragmatic hernia caused no further trouble, and her menstrual periods came without pain, swelling, or tension. Other long-standing problems also vanished, including recurrent pneumonia, the varicose veins in her legs, and the lumps and bumps on her back and breasts.

"Last winter I took up cross-country skiing and ice skating again," Diane reported in 1978. "I used to feel chilled all winter. Now I find pleasure at being outdoors in the cold. My attitude and my body have changed drastically, my entire life has changed for the better." In the six years since her recovery, Diane has become active in the East West Center in Toronto, teaching macrobiotic cooking and a more natural way of life to others.

Cervical Cancer: Donna Gail ━━━━━━━━━━━━━━━━━━

In 1969, twenty-seven-year-old Donna Gail of New Haven, Connecticut learned that she had cancer of the surface of her cervix. Several Pap smears, two biopsies, and a conization in which several layers of tissue around the cervix were scraped at Yale New Haven Community Hospital confirmed the diagnosis.

Prior to that time she had not paid much attention to her diet, and her favorite foods had been frozen sweets (including ice cream, cake, and candy bars), beef, macaroni, salt, tomato sauce, and cheese. She also drank about twenty cups of coffee a day. Concerned about her weight and health, Donna altered her diet considerably following discovery of the cancerous condition. She reduced the volume of her food consumption in general and reduced animal foods, including dairy food by about a third. She reduced her intake of refined flour, sugar, and sweets by 75 percent and tried to cut out all processed and artificial food.

In 1972 she learned about macrobiotics and came to hear me at a lecture at Rhode Island. The next day she decided to make whole grains the center of her diet and eliminated meat and dairy products entirely as well as strong sweets and raw food. "My diet became more balanced," she explained. "I now had a principle to follow. That was very important because I had never had any dietary principle, nor had I understood the idea of balance."

In 1975, after a period of difficulty in her life, her eating habits became irregular and the cervical problem returned. The gynecologist told her, "We have to do a biopsy. I am almost 100 percent sure you have cancer, and you need to have your reproductive organs removed." Donna returned the next day expecting him to tell her the biopsy had been positive. "No, you absolutely do not have cancer," the doctor reported. "You have an irritation. However, I still highly recommend that you have all of your organs removed as a preventive measure."

Donna refused and came to see me again for a consultation. I told her that she was consuming too many flour products and that even whole-wheat bread and baked products could contribute mucus to her system. Grains are preferably eaten in whole form, rather than as flour. Donna reduced her consumption of flour and flour products, and the irritation in her cervix went away.

A variety of other ailments also cleared up as her understanding and practice of macrobiotics improved. She experienced reserves of energy for the first time in years, and her fainting spells stopped.

Before, her menstrual period had also been debilitatingly painful. After two months following macrobiotic dietary principles, all pain disappeared. The flow had lightened and decreased from seven to five days. She had no more bloating before her period or soreness in her breasts. A scalp condition from which she suffered since childhood vanished, and her hemorrhoids went away.

There were other unexpected benefits as her way of life became more harmonious. "One of the most important changes I have been able to make since becoming macrobiotic," Donna confided, "involves my relationship with my father. Up until two years ago, I hadn't spoken with him since I was twelve years old. Now we communicate regularly and have discovered a great mutual respect and caring for one another."

Donna is now a licensed practical nurse (LPN). She has worked as a nutritional consultant on both the East and West coasts, and her experience in overcoming cancer has greatly benefited others.

Cystic Ovaries and Scar Tissue: Julie Hafer —————

I was very sick in August of 1982. I had lost weight gradually over the spring and summer, I was often tired, and I had frequent emotional upsets. But I really didn't see what was happening. Then, towards the end of August, my menstrual period was ten days long, and very, very heavy. I felt extremely weak. My back ached and my stomach was so sensitive it hurt when I walked. Lying on my back also hurt.

Frightened, I called the doctor, but he couldn't see me until the next week. Even though I was aching and flowing heavily, I forced myself to attend a macrobiotic cooking class at the Way of Life Center.

When I went to see the doctor, the first thing he did was to remove my IUD, which had been in for about a year. He said my tubes and ovaries felt scarred and he wanted to have a sonagram immediately. The test showed that my ovaries were cystic and my tubes were surrounded with massive scar tissue. The doctor wanted to admit me to the hospital immediately. Crying, I called home from his office and gave the news to my family.

Blood tests indicated that there was no infection, but my doctor felt that something about the results was not right. He put me on intravenous antibiotics for several days, and then I was scheduled for exploratory surgery.

The doctor told me that I might need a hysterectomy. This really upset me. I refused to sign the papers giving him permission to remove whatever he found. Then it was his turn to become agitated. He looked at me and asked, "Well, what if it is cancer?" I looked right back at him and said, "I want to know what it is, then I'll decide."

I will never forget the pressure I felt. This scene took place the evening before my surgery. The thought of cancer had never occurred to me. I felt frightened and alone. My nerves were already in poor condition; I cried uncontrollably. A nurse came in and tried to reassure me that a hysterectomy really wasn't so awful.

The doctor never did give my condition a name. He did say that it wasn't endometriosis. He said that my tubes were cystic, that the scar tissue was massive, and that he had extracted a milky looking fluid. He also said I had an infection going. I suspect that the IUD caused a low-grade infection for months.

The doctor said that he didn't think I could ever get pregnant. I already had three daughters from a former marriage, so this wasn't as bad as it might have been. Besides, I doubted that it was true.

After being discharged, I went again to the Way of Life Center, this time for more information on macrobiotics. I was very weak. I could cook, some. I ended up putting everything in the pressure cooker and eating that. I was the only one in the house eating this way, and this made it all the more difficult. I did manage to get the rest of the family to eat more grains and vegetables, however.

I continued to go to classes at the center, and the support of the people there made things easier.

I used a diaphram, but having grown accustomed to the IUD, often forgot to insert it. Besides, I remembered what the doctor had said. Four months after I started macrobiotics I was pregnant. My husband had been adopted, and the idea of having his first blood link was very special. We were both very happy.

I am glad that I was familiar with macrobiotics, if only in a general way, before I was hospitalized. My husband was very supportive when I told him I wanted to give it a try. I don't think I would have done it if he hadn't been. The people at the Way of Life Center were also extremely helpful. They were always there to offer encouragement and to provide information.

One final point: when I knew I was pregnant, I went to see the doctor one last time. He was suprised. He said he felt no scar tissue. And even though he acted as if he didn't think dietary changes had been responsible, he did say that it sounded like a diet he should be on.

Endometriosis: Tonia Gagne ─────────────────

In the early 1970s, nineteen-year-old Tonia Gagne was diagnosed as having endometriosis, a disease that results from an implantation of tissue within the walls of the uterus and around the ovaries and intestines. She had just had a baby, which she gave up for adoption, and soon after began to have a profuse vaginal discharge and agonizing cramps. Following two months in the hospital, she had her left ovary and Fallopian tube surgically removed. Doctors put her on hormonal therapy and prescribed Enovid-10. As a result of taking this pill three times a day for nine months, her hair began to fall out and her mental state, already fragile, deteriorated.

In 1973 Tonia went to live at the Zen Center in San Francisco, and meditation helped center her life. A friend introduced her to macrobiotics and the principles of ecological cooking. Nevertheless, Tonia, whose ancestry was partly Puerto Rican, was still attracted to some of the tropical food on which she grew up. "One of the things I loved was fried bananas," she said, looking back on this time in her life. "When I was told that if I wanted to practice macrobiotics correctly, I would have to give up fried bananas, I said, 'Oh no, not that.'" She included some brown rice, miso soup, and vegetables in her diet but continued to eat dairy food, sugar, and fried bananas. She went off Enovid-10, but her health continued to worsen.

In April 1976, Tonia returned to New England, and doctors at South Boston Community Center told her that the endometriosis had come back. Medical tests showed that she also had uterine cysts, and her right ovary had swollen to the size of a tennis ball. The doctors told her they would have to operate and she would never be able to have children again.

Tonia decided against the operation and moved into a macrobiotic study house where trained cooks prepared a special diet for her condition. Within three months on balanced food and no fried bananas, the cyst had disappeared. Over the next year her health improved, but the vaginal discharge persisted, and she still suffered from occasional cramps. In August 1977, Tonia and her new husband came to see me at the East West Foundation's summer program in Amherst.

"I sat down with Michio and he looked at my left hand and my left foot," she noted afterward. "He looked into my eyes and examined my face and then he said to me, 'You have no left ovary, right? Also, right ovary not so good, right? Also, tumor in your descending colon.' Then he looked at me and said, 'Maybe you have cancer.'"

I took out a piece of paper and drew a diagram describing the exact proportions of food she should be eating. I told her to eat 60 percent whole-cereal grains, the rest cooked vegetables, miso soup, various condiments, and to avoid all animal products, especially dairy food and meat. I told her to eliminate all oil, flour products, and fruits from her diet until her condition improved and to take regular hip baths in daikon leaves and to apply a plaster of taro potato over her reproductive organs to loosen the accumulation of fat and mucus.

"Within two weeks after I followed that diet," Tonia reported, "the pain subsided. I had a feeling of elation. My energy came back and a lot of worry was gone."

During the next two years, Tonia had to eat very strictly. Even the slightest deviation, such as an occasional peanut butter cookie or a carob brownie, would bring back the pain, cramps, and other symptoms of endometriosis. Gradually, however, she began to enjoy macrobiotic cooking and adjusted to living in a temperate climate without eating bananas and other tropical foods. About seven months after she began to practice the diet correctly, she became pregnant. Six weeks after giving birth to her son, Taran, she underwent a full examination by her physician. Medical tests showed no sign of endometriosis.

"Now I find myself much happier and more fulfilled," Tonia concluded several years after fully restoring her health. "Macrobiotics isn't any kind of religion or belief system. I had thought that macrobiotics would take the fun out of my life, but instead, I have learned to have more fun. I've learned balance. My life (and sense of enjoyment) is much simpler and much more fulfilling than I have ever felt."

In January 1981, Tonia gave birth to a second child by natural childbirth at her home and experienced no complications. For a woman who was told she would never have children again, Tonia has become a living example of faith in the healing powers of nature. A balanced diet is the birthright of us all. Sources: "Endometriosis and Tumor in the Colon," *The Cancer Prevention Diet* (Brookline, Mass.: East West Foundation, 1981, pp. 90–91), and Tom Monte, "Journey to Motherhood: Tonia's Truiumph Over Illness and Infertility," *East West Journal*, March 1982, pp. 44–48.

Endometriosis: Dawn Gilmour

When I was seventeen-years-old I went to the doctor with pain in my back and sides. I also had extremely painful menstruation which had gone on for several years. A blood test and urine samples were taken, but nothing could be found, and I was put on antibiotics and pain killers. In 1969, I went into the hospital for one month with nephritis.

Then, in 1972, after complaining for a number of years about the same pain and having been in the hospital four times for observation, I was told that my condition was probably psychosomatic. My doctors also told me that they would "open me up to keep me quiet," and when they did, they found that I had acute appendicitis and a cyst on the right ovary.

I never did feel right after that operation. I became very weak and continued going into the hospital for investigations, and was continually on antibiotics.

In 1976 it was discovered that I had endometriosis. I also had ovarian cysts and blocked Fallopian tubes. My surgeon, one of the leading female gynecologists in Scotland, tried to persuade me to have a hysterectomy. I was only twenty-four, and was told that with all of the trouble I had had, "it was just useless baggage." I really had to battle with the surgeon not to have the hysterectomy. During the operation my tubes were cut and "unblocked," and cysts and tissue from the endometriosis were removed. I was then given heat treatment because it was felt that I was not healing quickly enough. Large electric pads were placed on the ovary region. These pads conducted tremendous heat, and I stopped after four treatments because it was causing blisters on my skin and excessive bleeding.

I then went for a second opinion. The surgeon who I saw was shocked at my condition and could not believe that I was still walking around. I was sent immediately to the hospital for rest and observation. This new doctor said that heat treatment should not be used for my condition as it would accelerate the endometriosis. So in 1977, surgery was performed to remove the left Fallopian tube which had collapsed. Cysts were also removed from the ovaries.

I was then put on hormone treatments so as to suppress all menstruation, as this was believed to be a factor in spreading the endometriosis. One month after this operation I had a pelvic abscess and was rushed by ambulance to the hospital. They could not operate as it was too dangerous. I was placed in intensive care. I was given blood transfusions, could not urinate, and had tubes everywhere. The doctor did not think I would live. After two weeks the abscess burst and began to drain through the bowel. Little did I know that this would mean I would be running to the toilet up to nine times a day for the next month.

I stayed on the hormones for nine months and then decided to stop taking them. I was having severe headaches and pains in my kidneys, and had gone from 91 to 128 pounds. My heart felt very strained. I had no energy and looked like a walking balloon.

In 1978 I went back into the hospital for an investigation to see how things were going. I really felt no difference. It turned out that everything had accelerated and I was back to square one. The surgeon looked at me and said, "I don't know what to say."

During these years of illness I had tried many alternative approaches to healing, including acupuncture, homeopathy, herbs, and faith healing. I had also tried eating a vegetarian diet since 1972. Nothing seemed to make any long-term difference. I had also seen psychiatrists and was classed as a manic depressive.

I then met a friend who told me about macrobiotics. I decided to go to London to see Mr. Kushi. I felt I could not do any more damage by trying something else. I was so desperate to get well—to feel human again.

Mr. Kushi gave me certain dietary recommendations which I followed. I felt a difference within four days. Physically, I knew it was going to take a little time to get well, but the change in my mental attitude was so dramatic, so quick, I could hardly believe it. It was an overwhelming transformation for me, and my husband was thrilled with his "new wife."

Nine months later I went back to the Royal Infirmary for another internal examination. No endometriosis was found. My doctor, who had performed my previous surgery, thought that my recovery was unbelievable; he was so happy for me and encouraged me to continue on the macrobiotic diet as that seemed to be the thing that was changing my condition.

My last checkup was in September of 1981, just before I moved to Boston. I had an internal examination and Pap smear. Again, the results showed no problems.

I am so grateful to Mr. Kushi, to my husband who supported me continuously, and to all my friends for their support; without their compassion and encouragement things would have been so difficult. We must have this support, faith, and determination, and must realize that we are responsible for our own health and that we have the ability to change everything.

8. Our Future ━━━━━━━━━━

There is a Chinese expression, "May you live in interesting times," which has ambivalent overtimes. For some it is a curse, for others a blessing.

"Non-interesting" times exist when the pace of life is slower, great or cataclysmic events are not occurring, and life is more direct, simple, and stable. The pattern of life changes little throughout an individual's lifetime and what surrounds seems secure and dependable. It is during these times that one can find peace and live a more predictable and regular life.

On the other hand, "interesting" times represent a period of tremendous social change. These changes occur so rapidly that instead of stability there is constant upheaval and turmoil. Cataclysmic events become regular occurrences. Individual lives are subject to sudden change and great pressure. What is around us seems to change as rapidly as the scenery from the windows of a speeding car.

The result is the loss of traditional guidelines in individual, family, and social behavior. Nothing ever remains the same, but in interesting times the good old days were as recent as yesterday.

This definition suggests that we are living in interesting times—a period of intense and pervasive change and challenge. Either directly or indirectly, this challenge is aimed at our humanity—our health and happiness. We are being pushed in unknown directions with unknown consequences awaiting us.

During our lifetime we make many choices. But we will make the most important decision of our lives when we choose between the two divergent trends that characterize our age. One trend, impelled by the specter of sickness and ill health, is leading to an increasingly artificial lifestyle. Each major unit of human existence—the individual, the family, the social institutions including religion, education, and government—is being distorted by the impact of biological degeneration. Bewildered and powerless to act, these groups are abandoning their historic roles to science and technology. The result is disruption and chaos in society.

Suprisingly, the validity of this approach goes unquestioned. If it were effective, health-related problems would by now certainly be on the decline. As we have seen, this is simply not the case. Yet, instead of asking why, we await the newest remedies from the laboratory and the factory.

The complementary trend to this one of sickness and decline, is directed toward vibrant and natural health. It is characterized by harmony with nature in individual lifestyle—including diet—and the reorientation of the various aspects of society around this harmony. The goal is to eliminate the cause of ill health and to restore stability to society. The methods used to accomplish this are extremely simple. In fact, they are so simple that they are consistently overlooked by those caught in the trend towards complexity and artificiality.

For thousands of years humanity has thrived on a natural and harmonious way of life. Having met the test of time, this approach is practical beyond reproach. Technological solutions to the problems facing modern society are really quite new, most have been generated in the years since 1950. Despite exaggerated claims, they remain untested over the long term, and sadly ineffective in the short run. The importance of these major trends demands a more detailed examination.

Mechanical Response

Biological decline has generated two overlapping responses: the mechanization of the human body, and attempts to biologically alter the body's natural functions. The process of mechanization has resulted in industrialization and mass production. As mentioned earlier, various mechanical devices have been developed to save time, and to increase productivity and efficiency. The effects of industrialization have been pervasive. Modern society is a direct result of this process.

While this was going on in the workplace, mechanization was also being applied to the human body. Devices such as eye glasses, false teeth, crutches, braces, respirators, canes, and hearing aids provide mechanical assistance to an ailing body. Obviously, these things do not constitute a cure or an elimination of particular problems. They are stop-gap measures designed to enable individuals to function with some degree of normalcy. As our technology has become more complex, so have the devices used to support bodily functions.

Nothing reflects the symptomatic nature of this approach more than the fact that this field has exploded in recent decades. The health industry is one of the fastest growing sectors in our economy. Companies in the field are in fierce competition in the race to get new products to the marketplace. The promise of hundreds of millions of dollars awaits each new winner. As one commentator noted, there is an ongoing "medical arms race" between hospitals as they compete to provide state-of-the-art technology to attract patients.

What we fail to realize is that the necessity for such "crutches" implies a failure to prevent or to cure these problems. Instead, we have opted for ever more complex "band aids." This is reflected in the mechanization of the internal body. Devices are inserted into the body to replace diseased organs or body parts, or to alter basic biological processes.

According to conservative estimates, heart disease now strikes one of every four Americans, or twenty-five percent of the population. Faced with this challenge, our response has been to intensify our dependence on technology. Examples include the pacemaker, which regulates heart beat, and the development of the artifical heart. The human body, however, is not like an automobile, in which worn parts are replaced. Acting as if it were ignores the interaction of organs and systems, and body and mind.

Currently, about 36 million Americans suffer from arthritis; a degenerative disease that primarily strikes the body's joints. They become twisted and swollen with excruciating pain. Medications can provide temporary relief at best. In response, the replacement of a diseased hip joint with an artifical ball-and-socket device is a routine procedure. Joints for the knee, wrist, fingers and toes are either now in use or soon will be.

In the near future, it may be possible to replace other organs and body parts. Examples include an artifical kidney to filter our blood, or artifical lungs that mechanically duplicate the process of respiration.

In regard to the reproductive organs, there are mechanical devices for both males and females. For females, the insertion of the IUD or the diaphragm to prevent pregnancy represent mechanical interference with the natural process of reproduction. In men, there is an implantation device to mask the symptoms of impotence.

If present trends continue, the use of robots to perform tasks formerly done by humans will become pervasive. As the rate of degenerative disease increases, the use of sophisticated mechanical and automated parts based on robot technology will be applied to human beings. The result will be a new species, a combination of human and robot, or *hubot*, that is partly biological and partly mechanical. When this happens, we will have lost our biological integrity and severed our link to nature. We will no longer be children of God and nature, but the offspring of technology.

Biological Response

There is a biological parallel to this mechanical approach to illness. It involves the attempt to alter normal biological processes, including conception, pregnancy, and birth. It is being extended from the human being to the entire plant and animal kingdoms.

This trend began with attempts to change the chemistry of the body. Traditionally, mankind has used a variety of plant and animal products to treat various conditions. In the nineteenth century it became possible to isolate and extract specific substances from their natural sources. These chemical extracts became the foundation of modern medicine. In the twentieth century the production of these substances from synthetic sources began.

In 1953 researchers Francis Crick and James Watson unraveled the pattern of DNA, making it possible to chart the inner mechanism of the cell. The ability to alter basic biological processes emerged, and medicine's focus narrowed to the cellular level.

A preliminary part of this trend has been the transplanting of biological organs. This began with heart transplants from animal to human, and was soon followed by organ transplants from human to human. Research is now underway to grow replacement organs in a laboratory.

Because of the alarming increase of infertility cases, high technology is now being applied to reproductive processes. Artificial insemination, which had been used on animals for breeding purposes, was refined and applied to human beings. The union of sperm and egg outside the body, known as in vitro fertilization, was a further refinement. Later, because of the low success rate and the difficulty involved in retrieving and implanting eggs, improvements were made in this process. A number of eggs were removed from a woman's ovary. They were then fertilized and the extra ones were frozen to be used if initial attempts at pregnancy failed.

The birth of the first frozen embryo occurred in March 1984, by emergency Caesarean section in Melbourn, Australia. The parent's fertilized egg had been frozen for two months before being thawed and implanted.

There are no medical or scientific guidelines to assess the effects of these technologies on human beings. At best, the approach is a wait and see attitude. The macrobiotic principles, however, gives us practical insight into what is going on and what can be expected.

Fertilization outside the body represents a biological reversal from human beings to aquatic creatures. During the process of evolution, the external fertilization of lower animals evolved into internal fertilization and gestation in higher animals.

Because external fertilization is not a natural characteristic in human beings, various technological devices are needed to accomplish what can only be described as a de-evolutionary process. A baby born from this method is greatly weakened. Individually, the vitality of sperm and egg cells is diminished when they are removed from their natural environment. And of course, if left unattended, they soon die.

This is a critical point because upon fertilization, the egg and sperm become the foundation of our two most basic systems, the digestive and nervous systems. This occurs about twenty-four hours after conception when the fertilized ovum divides into two cells. In another twelve hours these two will divide into four cells. This division continues roughly every twelve hours, and correlates to the rotation of the earth. Approximately every twelve hours, the two halves of the twenty-four-hour daily cycle—day and night—alternate. This pattern reflects the interaction of Heaven's and Earth's force on our planet.

The fertilized ovum spins on its axis and divides in response to the same energy pattern that moves the earth. This basic pattern of division controls growth in the plant kingdom where growth can be viewed as the increase in cellular structure and the specialization of cell groups such as seeds, roots, stems, branches, flowers, and fruit.

In the newly fertilized ovum, this process of division sets the foundation for the various systems, and from these building blocks, the organs develop. The quality, strength, and vitality of each organ and each system is greatly affected if fertilization takes place outside the female body.

During intercourse, as the man's sperm are deposited in the vagina, a process of natural selection goes on. A relatively few sperm out of the millions ejaculated, survive the journey through the female reproductive tract, and only one fertilizes an egg. It is not likely that the strongest sperm will be chosen for use in the various fertility technologies.

The union of egg and sperm takes place under specific conditions, including a warm, moist, dark environment, with slightly higher pressure than the external environment. Human biological secretions occur in specific amounts and at precise moments. When conception and early cell division occur outside the womb, these influences are lost.

The mother's body supplies an intensive charge of energy to the rapidly dividing fetus. We have already seen how Heaven's and Earth's force create a primary channel of energy flow in the human body. Fetal development unfolds within one of the major energy centers on this channel. In external fertilization, the crucial early stages of cell division take place without this energy.

When fertilized eggs are frozen, the whole process of growth and development is interrupted. Cell division stops and the strength and vitality of all systems and organs is further diminished. Children born from such methods could require specialized environments to survive. They may be something like greenhouse flowers, which may grow big and beautiful in a controlled environment, but which have lost their ability to adapt and survive in the natural environment. The loss of strength and vitality signifies the loss of adaptability.

Future Visions

With advances in DNA research, the process of mapping various genes is under way. The correlation between the location of a gene on a DNA strand and what it controls in the body is being charted. In the future, defective or unwanted genes will be removed and new, "desirable" genes implanted. In the years ahead, we will witness an increasing ability to select the characteristics most desirable in a child.

One of the most startling concepts in futuristic technology is the artifical womb. After in vitro fertilization, the ovum will be placed in a special container where it will presumably develop into a human infant. The environment will be computor controlled to simulate the condition of a woman's uterus during pregnancy. This will remove the burden of childbearing from women. There is speculation on the possibility of designing artificial sperm and egg cells, that would then be united and used in the artificial womb.

At the extreme, there could be a mating of mechanical and biological trends. This could include the implantation of various computer chips into the body by means of an artificial cell to correct various physical and mental disorders. The result would be a biotronic being or *biotron*, a biological, electronic being.

Vast numbers of biotrons, of lower intelligence and programmed to do certain tasks, could be employed as a servant force, a worker force, or even a police and military force in future society. Please do not make the mistake of thinking that all of this is science fiction. It most certainly is not. These developments are well under way, and the technological ability to accomplish them is being laid down here and now. We do indeed live in interesting times.

These mechanical and biological approaches are being pursued for the following reasons:

1. The widespread incidence of degenerative disease.
2. The inability to prevent or satisfactorily treat these degenerative disorders.
3. The total lack of an overall framework that explains the diverse problems in modern society.

The Health Response ─────────────────────────

We have seen how the epidemic of declining health in modern societies has generated a two-pronged, artifical response in a desperate attempt to, if not change, at least compensate. In nature an extreme state cannot exist in isolation. The opposite will emerge to create balance.

The complementary trend emerging in modern society is the movement toward a more natural way of life. This includes the concept of assuming responsibility for one's health, and realizing the tremendous influence our lifestyle, and in particular our way of eating, has on our total self. As a mirror image of the trend toward declining health, this opposite trend also has two aspects.

The first includes various approaches that can be categorized under the heading of non-principled health. This category is based on the assumption that one particular or partial aspect can insure health. Examples include:

1.   Vitamin enthusiasts. The vitamin enthusiasts feel that the body is made up of varying amounts of different chemical substances and that health comes from taking regular and sometimes mega amounts of them. This line of thinking holds that food—for various reasons— is inadequately supplied, thus the necessity for supplementation. In the extreme, there is the tendency to think that taking scientifically designed nutritional pills is superior to eating.

2.   Exercise enthusiasts. There is a certain train of thought that supposes that vigorous daily physical activity can negate the effects of an imbalanced diet by "burning" out any excess or poisons. In some instances there is a combination of exercise and a particular dietary orientation to enhance the effectiveness of exercise.

3.   Food faddists. Food faddists tend to believe in the superior merits of one particular food that can insure total health. Examples include honey, yogurt, and any of a variety of special juices. By eating huge amounts of this food, or by eating it exclusively, they believe that health can be maintained.

4.   Analytical approach. People using the analytical approach to health see food as a combination of isolated elements. They reason that by taking these elements in proportions found in the body they can ensure health.

Each of these approaches has some merit. First, they recognize the concept of self-health and the necessity for accepting responsibility for our lives. Secondly, they recognize the relationship between diet and/or lifestyle and health.

Both of these factors reflect shifts in the thinking among the medical and scientific community. Increasingly, studies are pointing to the link between health and diet and lifestyle. And these findings are finding their way into reports and recommendations of health-related institutions.

However, because these approaches use partial methods, and because they lack the comprehensive understanding needed to create overall well-being, their results are necessarily partial. They cannot protect us from sickness, nor can they provide for our continual development on all levels.

Macrobiotics

The second major aspect of the trend towards health is macrobiotics. Based on universal principles, macrobiotics enables us to create harmony in our own lives, and between ourselves and life at large. While representing a comprehensive approach to diet and lifestyle, macrobiotics offers us the tools to work with social and global issues as well. This opportunity is open to anyone who choses to use it.

Guidelines for the Future

For the past two to three hundred years, progress has been measured in terms of mankind's ability to construct devices that increase efficiency and comfort, and that reduces misery and misery. Science has played a dominant role in this area. It has increased human knowledge with its at times stunning discoveries. The business world has brought the results of these discoveries to the average person in a practical way.

Unfortunately, not all of these discoveries have been beneficial to humanity or to the planet. And yet it has been only very recently that we have begun to question the wisdom, utility, and long-term benefits of unquestioningly accepting the latest scientific or technological innovation.

How we respond to reproductive disorders and infertility reflects our choice in regard to the divergent trends mentioned earlier. Do we want a future in which technology becomes a normal part of reproduction. And do we want to accept the possibility of artificially created life. Or do we want to return to normal, natural health. The following guidelines will help clarify our position:

1. Does our choice increase natural health and happiness for the individual, family, society, and hence the world.
2. Does our choice foster a closer union with nature or does it increase separation.
3. Does our choice promote harmony and peace.
4. Does our choice benefit all of humanity or only a few.

Conclusions

The energies of Heaven and Earth create and sustain us. Sickness is a sign that these energies are not flowing smoothly and normally through our body. This is a result of our own way of life, not because of any deficiency in Heaven's and Earth's force.

For real healing to occur, we must accept responsibility for our condition. This starts with the recognition that we are out of harmony with the larger forces of nature; that we are violating the universal principles of nature. No matter how long we have been ill, the forces of life are there for us to use. They are available to everyone. No matter how we were conceived, how we were born, and how we have lived up to this point, the forces of life are freely available to everyone.

For all those who have been born of various birth technologies this is true; for everyone who is sick this is true; and for anyone facing emotional or mental conflict it is true. Life supports life, if we are willing to allow it to do so.

Resources ━━━━━━━━━━━━━━━━━━━━━━

Macrobiotics International in Boston and its major educational centers in the United States, Canada, and around the world offer ongoing classes for the general public in macrobiotic cooking and traditional food preparation and natural processing. They also offer instruction in Oriental medicine, shiatsu massage, pregnancy and natural child care, yoga, meditation, science, culture and the arts, and world peace and world government activities. Macrobiotics International Educational Centers also provide way of life guidance services with trained and certified consultants, make referrals to professional health care associates, and cooperate in research and food programs in hospitals, medical schools, prisons, drug rehabilitation clinics, nursing homes, and other institutions. In scores of other cities and communities, there are smaller Macrobiotics International learning centers, residential centers, and information centers offering some classes and services.

Most of the foods mentioned in this book are available at natural food stores, selected health food stores, and a growing number of supermarkets around the world. Macrobiotic specialty items are also available by mail order from various distributors and retailers.

Please contact Macrobiotics International in Boston or other national centers listed below for information on regional and local activities in your area, as well as whole foods outlets and mail order sources.

Global Headquarters
Macrobiotics International
Box 568
Brookline, Mass. 02147
617-738-0045

Australia
Australian Macrobiotic
  Association
1 Carlton St., Prahran
Melbourne, 3181
Australia
03-529-1620

Belgium
Oost West Centrum
  Kushi Institute
Consciencestraat 48
Antwerpen, 2000
Belgium
03-230-13-82

Bermuda
Macrobiotic Center
  of Bermuda
In-The-Lee, Deepwood
  Drive Fairyland
Pembroke, Bermuda
809-29-5-2275

Britain
Community Health
  Foundation
188-194 Old Street
London, ECIV 9BP
England
01-251-4076

Canada
861 Queen Street
Toronto, Ontario
M6J IC4, Canada

France
Le Grain Sauvage
  Macrobiotic
  Association
15 Rue Letellier, 75015
Paris, France
33-1-828-4773

Germany
Ost West Zentrum
Eppendorfer
 Marktplatz
13 D-2000, Hamburg 20
040–47–27–50

Holland
Oost West Centrum
 Kushi Institute
Achtergracht 17
1017 WL Amsterdam
Holland
020–240–203

Hong Kong
Conduit RD 41A
Rome CT. 8D Hong
 Kong, Hong Kong
5–495–268

Israel
24 Amos Street
Tel Aviv, Israel
442979

Italy
Fondazione Est Ovest
Via de'Serragli 4
50124 Florence, Italy

Japan
Macrobiotics—Tokyo
20–9 Higashi Mine
Ota-ku, Tokyo 146
Japan
03–753–9216

Lebanon
Mary Naccour
Couvent St. Elie
Box 323 Antelias
Beirut, Lebanon

Norway
East West Center
Frydenlundsgt 2 0169
Oslo 1, Norway
02–60–47–79

Portugal
Unimave
Rua Mouzinha da
 Silveira 25, 1200
Lisbon, Portugal
1–557–362

Switzerland
Ost West Zentrum
Postfach 2502, Bern
3001 Switzerland
031–25–65–40

United Arab Emirates
Box 4943 SATWA
Dubai, United Arab
 Emirates
040440–031
 (national)
97–1–44–4–0031
 (international)

United Nations
United Nations
 Macrobiotics Society
c/o Katsuhide Kitatani
U.N. Development
 Programme
1 United Nations
Plaza, New York
N. Y. 10017
212–906–5844

United States
Kushi Institute
17 Station Street
Brookline, Mass.
02147
617–738–0045

Bibliography

Macrobiotic Health Education Series

Kushi, Michio. *A Natural Approach: Allergies*. Edited by Mark Mead and John D. Mann. Tokyo: Japan Publications, Inc., 1985.
————. *A Natural Approach: Diabetes and Hypoglycemia*. Edited by John D. Mann. Tokyo: Japan Publications, Inc., 1985.

Macrobiotic Food and Cooking Series

Kushi, Aveline. *Cooking for Health: Allergies*. Edited by Rosalind Rhodes. Tokyo: Japan Publications, Inc., 1985.
————. *Cooking for Health: Diabetes and Hypoglycemia*. Edited by Rosalind Rhodes. Tokyo: Japan Publications, Inc., 1985.

Cookbooks

Aihara, Cornellia. *Macrobiotic Kitchen*. Tokyo: Japan Publications, Inc., 1983.
————. *The Do of Cooking*, Chico. Calif.: George Ohsawa Macrobiotic Foundation, 1972.
Esko, Edward and Wendy. *Macrobiotic Cooking for Everyone*. Tokyo: Japan Publications, Inc., 1980.
Esko, Wendy. *Introducing Macrobiotic Cooking*. Tokyo: Japan Publications, Inc., 1978.
Estella, Mary. *Natural Foods Cookbook: Vegetarian Dairy-free Cuisine*. Tokyo: Japan Publications, Inc., 1985.
Kushi, Aveline. *How to Cook with Miso*. Tokyo: Japan Publications, Inc., 1978.
Kushi, Aveline, with Alex Jack. *Aveline Kushi's Complete Guide to Macrobiotic Cooking for Health, Harmony, and Peace*. N. Y.: Warner Publishing Co., 1984.
Kushi, Aveline, with Wendy Esko. *The Changing Seasons Macrobiotic Cookbook*. Wayne, N. J.: Avery Publishing Group, 1984.
Ohsawa, Lima. *Macrobiotic Cuisine*. Tokyo: Japan Publications, Inc., 1984.

Other Macrobiotic or Related Books

Aihara, Herman. *Basic Macrobiotics*. Tokyo: Japan Publications, Inc., 1985.
Brown, Virginia, with Susan Stayman. *Macrobiotic Miracle: How a Vermont Family Overcame Cancer*. Tokyo: Japan Publications, Inc., 1985.
Dufty, William. *Sugar Blues*. New York: Warner, 1975.
Heidenry, Carolyn. *An Introduction to Macrobiotics: A Beginner's Guide to the Natural Way of Health*. Brookline Mass.: Aladdin Press, 1984.
————. *Making the Transition to a Macrobiotic Diet*. Brookline, Mass.: Aladdin Press, 1984.
Ineson, Rev. John. *The Way of Life: Macrobiotics and the Spirit of Chris-

tianity. Tokyo: Japan Publications, Inc., 1985.

Kohler, Jean and Mary Alice. *Healing Miracles from Macrobiotics*. West Nyack, N.Y.: Parker, 1979.

Kotzsch, Ronald E. *Macrobiotics: Yesterday and Today*. Tokyo: Japan Publications, Inc., 1985.

Kushi, Aveline. *Lessons of Day and Night*. Wayne, N. J.: Avery Publishing Group, 1984.

Kushi, Michio. *The Book of Dō-In: Exercise for Physical and Spiritual Development*. Tokyo: Japan Publications, Inc., 1979.

Kushi, Michio. *The Book of Macrobiotics* (Revised edition), Tokyo: Japan Publications, Inc., 1987.

———. *Cancer and Heart Disease: The Macrobiotic Approach to Degenerative Disorders* (Revised edition), Tokyo: Japan Publications, Inc., 1985.

———. *The Era of Humanity*. Edited by Sherman Goldman. Brookline, Mass.: East West Journal, 1980.

———. *How to See Your Health: The Book of Oriental Diagnosis*. Tokyo: Japan Publications, Inc., 1980.

———. *Macrobiotic Home Remedies*. Edited by Marc Van Cauwenberghe. Tokyo: Japan Publications, Inc., 1985.

———. *Natural Healing through Macrobiotics*. Tokyo: Japan Publications, Inc., 1987.

———. *Your Face Never Lies*. Wayne, N.J.: Avery Publishing Group, 1983.

Kushi, Michio and Aveline. *Macrobiotic Pregnancy and Care of the Newborn*. Tokyo: Japan Publications, Inc., 1984.

———. *Macrobiotic Child Care & Family Health*. Tokyo: Japan Publications, Inc., 1986.

Kushi, Michio, with Alex Jack. *The Cancer Prevention Diet*. N. Y.: St. Martin's Press, 1983.

———. *Diet for a Strong Heart: Michio Kushi's Macrobiotic Dietary Guidelines for the Prevention of High Blood Pressure, Heart Attack, and Stroke*. New York: St. Martin's Press, 1985.

Kushi, Michio and the East West Foundation. *Cancer and Heart Disease: The Macrobiotic Approach to Degenerative Disorders*. Edited by Edward Esko. Tokyo: Japan Publications, Inc., 1982.

Mendelsohn, Robert, S. *Confessions of a Medical Heretic*. Chicago: Contemporary Books, 1979.

———. *Male Practice*. Chicago: Contemporary Books, 1980.

Nussbaum, Elaine, *Recovery: From Cancer to Health Through Macrobiotics*. Tokyo: Japan Publications, Inc., 1985.

Ohsawa, George. *Cancer and the Philosophy of the Far East*. Oroville, Calif.: George Ohsawa Macrobiotic Foundation, 1971.

Ohsawa, George, with William, Dufty. *You Are All Sanpaku*. N. Y.: University Books, 1965.

Sattilaro, Anthony, with Tom Monte. *Recalled by Life: The Story of My Recovery from Cancer*. Boston: Houghton-Mifflin, 1982.

Tara, William. *Macrobiotics and Human Behavior*. Tokyo: Japan Publications, Inc., 1985.

Index ━━━━━━━━━━